Psychobabble

Psychobabble

**VIRAL MENTAL HEALTH MYTHS
& THE TRUTHS TO SET YOU FREE**

Joe Nucci, LPC

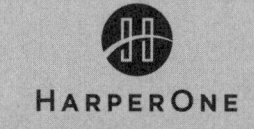

HarperOne
An Imprint of HarperCollins*Publishers*

Without limiting the exclusive rights of any author, contributor or the publisher of this publication, any unauthorized use of this publication to train generative artificial intelligence (AI) technologies is expressly prohibited. HarperCollins also exercise their rights under Article 4(3) of the Digital Single Market Directive 2019/790 and expressly reserve this publication from the text and data mining exception.

This book contains advice and information relating to health care. It should be used to supplement rather than replace the advice of your doctor or another trained health professional. If you know or suspect you have a health problem, it is recommended that you seek your physician's advice before embarking on any medical program or treatment. All efforts have been made to assure the accuracy of the information contained in this book as of the date of publication. This publisher and the author disclaim liability for any medical outcomes that may occur as a result of applying the methods suggested in this book.

The names and identifying characteristics of some individuals in this book have been changed to protect their privacy.

PSYCHOBABBLE. Copyright © 2025 by Joseph Nucci. All rights reserved. Printed in the United States of America. No part of this book may be used or reproduced in any manner whatsoever without written permission except in the case of brief quotations embodied in critical articles and reviews. For information, address HarperCollins Publishers, 195 Broadway, New York, NY 10007. In Europe, HarperCollins Publishers, Macken House, 39/40 Mayor Street Upper, Dublin 1, D01 C9W8, Ireland.

HarperCollins books may be purchased for educational, business, or sales promotional use. For information, please email the Special Markets Department at SPsales@harpercollins.com.

harpercollins.com

FIRST EDITION

Designed by Yvonne Chan

Library of Congress Cataloging-in-Publication Data has been applied for.

ISBN 978-0-06-342462-3
ISBN 978-0-06-347918-0 (ANZ)

25 26 27 28 29 LBC 5 4 3 2 1

This book is written in loving memory of my dad,
Joseph Anthony Nucci (1964–2005).

It is dedicated to all those who are grieving
or dealing with other inescapable problems of living.
You are not alone.

Contents

Introduction: The Tower of Psychobabble — 1

Part I—Freudian Fantasies: Common Myths About Mental Health and Psychology

Myth #1: "Everyone Should Go to Therapy" — 11
Myth #2: "Analyzing Your Thoughts Is Always Good for You" — 16
Myth #3: "Expressing Your Feelings Is Valid" — 22
Myth #4: "You Were Totally Projecting When That Happened" — 27
Myth #5: "Personality Frameworks Are Reductive, Inaccurate, and Not Helpful" — 33
Myth #6: "Hurt People Hurt People" — 38

Part II—DSM Mayhem: Common Myths About Mental Health Diagnoses

Myth #7: "Receiving a Diagnosis Is Terrible" — 45
Myth #8: "Mental Health Diagnoses Are Just Made-Up" — 50
Myth #9: "Your Diagnosis Is Your Identity" — 55
Myth #10: "You Can Diagnose Yourself" — 61

Contents

Part III—Clinical Cacophony: Common Myths About Popularly Misused Therapy Terms

Myth #11: "Everyone Gets Depressed and Anxious" — 71
Myth #12: "The Reason You Can't Focus Is ADHD" — 78
Myth #13: "Mindfulness Is Good for Everyone" — 84
Myth #14: "Your Awkward Friend Is Neurodivergent" — 88
Myth #15: "That Person Is a Psychopath" — 94
Myth #16: "Boundaries Are Just Preferences" — 99
Myth #17: "People Gaslight You When They Disagree" — 104
Myth #18: "Your Ex Is Definitely a Narcissist" — 112
Myth #19: "I Am a People Pleaser Because I Defer to You" — 121

Part IV—Trauma Drama: Common Myths About Trauma

Myth #20: "Everyone Has Trauma" — 129
Myth #21: "Trauma Is the Same Thing as Grief" — 135
Myth #22: "Disciplining Your Child Will Cause Trauma" — 140
Myth #23: "Your Trauma Made You an Empath" — 145
Myth #24: "Questioning Trauma Discourse Harms Survivors" — 150

Part V—Social Schisms: Common Myths About Mental Health and Society

Myth #25: "Your Mental Illness Is a Systemic Problem" — 159
Myth #26: "People Aren't Evil, They're Just Mentally Ill" — 164
Myth #27: "Mental Health Education Is Always Beneficial" — 169
Myth #28: "Psychotherapy Is the Only Way to Improve Your Mental Well-Being" — 176

Contents

Myth #29: "Party Animals Have Issues"   181
Myth #30: "Therapy Is Not Political"   188

Part VI—Shrink Secrets: Common Myths About Therapists

Myth #31: "Therapists Treat Clients, Not Patients"   201
Myth #32: "Therapists Should Never Give Advice"   204
Myth #33: "Therapists Psychoanalyze Everyone They Meet"   209
Myth #34: "Shrinks Are Crazier than Their Patients"   215
Myth #35: "Therapists Never Talk About Themselves with Patients"   220

Part VII—Relational Ruckus: Common Myths That Hurt Your Relationships

Myth #36: "Your Date Is Love-Bombing You"   227
Myth #37: "Freak in the Head, Freak in the Bed"   234
Myth #38: "The More Emotional Intimacy, the Better"   240
Myth #39: "Therapy Will Make You Ready for a Relationship"   246
Myth #40: "Using Therapeutic Language Makes You Emotionally Intelligent"   255

Acknowledgments   263
Notes   267

Introduction
The Tower of Psychobabble

The speed at which talking about mental health has gone from taboo to commonplace is unprecedented. Just a few decades ago, admitting that you struggled with depression, anxiety, obsessive-compulsive disorder (OCD), or any other mental health concern would constitute a serious social liability. People who sought out therapy risked being labeled crazy or psycho; they might be thought of as head cases and might even be considered dangerous. Today, however, speaking openly about mental health struggles is considered a sign of authenticity and personal strength.

Unlike other contentious topics in today's society, mental health appears to have shirked all manner of proscription. Mental health is a topic at dinnertime and even in the workplace. It's portrayed in movies and on television, openly discussed on podcasts and cable news channels. On social media, celebrities, politicians, professional athletes, and an army of ordinary people routinely discuss the details of their mental health in public spaces without fear of social retribution. In fact, the opposite is true. Mental health influencers stand to gain huge followings, make money, land book deals, and share their knowledge with millions of people. Jeff Guenther, better known as @therapyjeff on social media, once gave an interview in which he said he made almost a million dollars in one year from merchandise, brand deals, and direct subscriptions.[1] If I am being honest, I landed this book deal partly because of my own social media following.

There are still some cultures and subcultures in which discussions about mental health seemingly do not exist or are considered private, unsuitable for public airing. But throughout the Western world today, enough people speak openly about mental health to substantiate a *mental health culture*. Put simply, mental health culture consists of the people who talk about mental health and therefore influence the public's beliefs, values, practices, and corresponding systems of language in relation to mental health.

While everyone is talking about mental health, not everyone is *qualified* to do so. Sometimes mental health content creators are credentialed academics or professional clinicians like me. Like many creators, I practice psychotherapy and help people with mental health concerns. But frequently, the content creators doling out viral advice online are *mental health enthusiasts*, who enjoy talking about therapy-related topics or sharing stories about their mental health journeys but lack actual credentials, training, and clinical experience. And herein lies a serious problem.

Many professionals in this field worked tirelessly to shake off the taboo that overshadowed mental health for decades. But today, mental health is not just destigmatized—it's popularized. While this shift undoubtedly has some benefits, it also has many downsides. The popularization of mental health terminology has given rise to an army of armchair experts who regularly speak on the topic and—knowingly or unknowingly—misuse psychological jargon. They spread misinformation and often inflict a lot of damage in the process.

Given the sharp, unexpected, and potentially hazardous rise

in mental health culture, we need to talk about how we talk about mental health. We need to separate fact from fiction and folklore, but the problem is not just about misconceptions and misinformation. It's important to address terms that seemingly pop up out of nowhere and define what they *actually* mean and what they do *not* mean. We need to discuss the potentially harmful consequences that arise from misused terms and other kinds of misinformation. This conversation is not only necessary—it is long overdue.

Much of the most popular mental health content on the internet and social media today can be categorized as *psychobabble*—a fancy word that describes a form of communication that utilizes psychological language to create an *impression* of authority, truth, or plausibility. The root *psycho* refers to psychology or the study of the mind, and it's worth noting that *psycho* is derived from the Latin word *psyche*, meaning "of the spirit." The word *babble* is derived from a mid-thirteenth-century word *babeln*, which means "to utter words indistinctly, like a baby." Psychobabble is what often results when uncredentialed social media influencers (mis)use therapy-speak and mental health terminology.

The word *babble* is also a pun on the ancient tale of the Tower of Babel, though there is no known formal connection between the two. The story is most famously found in the book of Genesis in the Hebrew Bible, but the story has representations in different myths across cultures and history, with Sumerian, Assyrian, Greek, Roman, African, and Mexican parallels. You might call it a meta-myth, a cultural story that transcends historical and cultural divides.

While the story has various interpretations and translations, it generally goes as follows:

The whole Earth and everyone on the Earth spoke the same language, used the same words, and understood one another clearly. Then the people of the Earth, out of their hubris, decided to build a tall structure that would reach up to the heavens. But God, seeing this effort, decided to make everyone speak in different languages so they could not understand one another, and they were unable to finish building their tower. This incomplete structure was called the Tower of Babel.

Although myths and fables may not be historically factual, they are often valuable in that they reveal something about reality. So what can the story of the Tower of Babel reveal to us? First, it's warning us to have humility in our endeavors. Nothing human-made can ever truly reach the heavens, because we are and will always remain mere mortals.

This lesson is apropos for those of us who work in mental health. Nothing can truly erase life's negative qualities, and therapy has its limitations. No mental health therapist, no pill, no concept or turn of phrase can completely erase problems of living or fully explain life's hardships. Although some traditional interpretations of the Tower of Babel story teach that God stopped the structure from being built in order to punish the builders, I'm not so sure. I think it's possible that the motivation was love. After all, the road to hell is paved with good intentions; sometimes, you have to stop people, however well-meaning they are, from harming themselves and others. Perhaps, in the myth, God was stopping people from hurting themselves in ways they could not understand.

The Tower of Babel myth also stresses the importance of being on the same page when undertaking a daunting task. Whether you're building a tower to the heavens or building out mental health culture, it's helpful to speak the same language. We have to use a shared vocabulary with generally agreed-upon definitions and propagate concepts with a collectively understood scope. If people use the word *trauma* too broadly, to mean different things—as many often do now—then this vagueness will impact everything from individual therapy to the way people conduct and interpret trauma research. If people start expanding the definition of mental illness to cover basically every negative aspect of human existence—as they often do now—mental health will eventually become meaningless. If everything is mental health, then nothing is mental health. Words have meaning, and meanings matter.

Mental health culture is a structure worth building together. More people deserve therapy than currently get it. Mental health concerns harm not just individuals but also society at large. Untreated mental illness costs the US economy over $280 billion every year.[2] According to the US Department of Justice, around 50 percent of those in jail and prison are believed to have a mental illness.[3] We are a long way off from having a world where everyone who needs adequate mental health care receives it.

In my view, all progress to be made is downstream from culture. All systemic mental health progress depends on how we talk about mental health. Unless clinicians, researchers, writers, content creators, and all the people who make up mental health culture can begin to speak the same language, we will never successfully shape a sufficient mental health culture. If we cannot manage this situation, we will become like those who attempted to build the Tower of Babel, unable to speak with one another and ultimately leaving the project unfinished. Even worse, people like you will continue to encounter myths and misinformation online, putting you at risk of making impactful life and health care decisions based on information that is incorrect or only partially true.

I wrote *Psychobabble* to help you learn to identify the most common mental health myths circulated on the internet and social media—and to replace these myths with truths that will liberate you to make informed decisions about your own mental health and live a better life. Rather than simply recount facts, I'll introduce you to mental health concerns that I have treated in my private practice to demonstrate the most essential points about psychology and the treatment of mental illness. While every story comes from real experience, I have fictionalized identifying details to protect the confidentiality of the patients. In obscuring these details, I was careful to honor the core lessons of their experience in order to get at something essential and true about mental health treatment. As Albert Camus said, "Fiction is the lie we use to tell the truth." If you notice similarities between the stories that follow and your own, I hope you take comfort in knowing that there is something very human and universal about all these experiences. I also hope that finding these similarities helps you to feel less alone and more connected to the world around you. The central promise of mental health culture is exactly that: the potential to feel less alone. Mental health is about feeling more aware, more connected, and more understanding of your life, your relationships, and your inner world. When people misuse mental health terms or propagate misinformation, the result can be that you feel less aware, less connected, and less understanding.

The goal of this project is not to create a world where

everyone—therapists and patients alike—totally agrees on every matter related to mental health. Succeeding at such a task would be impossible. Even professional clinicians like me often disagree on what constitutes sound mental health advice. Within the mental health field and through ongoing conversations among clinicians, we're learning more day by day. As a result, there are deep philosophical disagreements among professionals in the field, and these disagreements fuel debates that propel us toward the truth. Instead, my goal is more modest: to dispel the most popular myths, identify the most destructive misinformation, and clarify the widely accepted meanings of often misused terms. Whenever different philosophical approaches can be taken, I will do my best to highlight the different perspectives and consider the pros and cons. That way, regardless of who you are, you can more skillfully navigate all the psychobabble you encounter on your own mental health journey.

I am grateful we live in a time when mental health is becoming more destigmatized, and I hope to help build a world where people view mental health concerns, such as post-traumatic stress disorder, as just as normal as other medical issues, like diabetes—a world where emotional regulation is as revered as an insulin shot. But the normalization of mental health must be accompanied by education and accountability. And that effort begins, right here, right now, by talking about how we talk about mental health, together.

Part I

Freudian Fantasies: Common Myths About Mental Health and Psychology

Myth #1: "Everyone Should Go to Therapy"

In her book *I Like You Just the Way I Am*, author Jenny Mollen says, "There are two types of people in the world: Those who think everyone needs therapy, and those who have never been."[1] Even a cursory scan of the internet and social media will tell you that Mollen is onto something.

The idea that everyone should have a therapist with whom they regularly meet is usually a well-intentioned belief. As a licensed and practicing psychotherapist, I often meet with a patient who is entering therapy for the very first time, and I have the privilege of witnessing their eyes light up with wonder at the level of self-knowledge they attain from doing "the work." Understandably, they then wish for everyone they know to have a similar experience. Unfortunately, the belief that absolutely everyone needs psychotherapy doesn't quite hold up to scrutiny. It's just not that simple. While it is true that almost anyone can benefit from therapy—assuming the therapist is ethical and competent—it is also true that not everyone requires therapy.

I came to this realization on the first day of my internship in graduate school when I was training to become a psychotherapist. When you begin seeing patients under clinical supervision, you're typically assigned only one or two at a time so you can find your footing. My first patient, Abby, had no observable mental health concerns. She sought therapy because she was curious about whether she had anxiety. I treated her for about a year, and we did really great work together. By the end of her treatment, Abby was a more self-aware, less self-conscious person who was living a more aligned life. But here's the truth: Abby would've been fine without therapy. She was smart and emotionally intelligent, and I am confident that she could have figured out her problems on her own, without my help. Our work together likely helped accelerate that process, but there is a big difference between a need and a benefit.

By contrast, Bill, my second patient, arrived with multiple diagnoses listed on his intake form. He was an hour late to his first session, and appointments at this clinic were only forty-five minutes long. Even though Bill missed his session, he was desperate to be seen by someone anyway. He arrived disheveled and emotionally dysregulated, and he had a hard time articulating his internal experience with words. I saw him for more than a year, and during that time, we discovered that his bipolar diagnosis (which he originally received from a previous practitioner) was likely a misdiagnosis. Instead, he had severe attention deficit hyperactivity disorder (ADHD) and a substantial history of trauma. I referred him to a psychiatrist, and after his medication was adjusted and he went through trauma therapy, he experienced a lot of symptom relief. When my internship ended, I eventually handed him off to another therapist at the clinic to continue treatment. In Bill's case—unlike Abby's situation—I do not think it's fair to say that he would've been fine without mental health treatment. These two patient vignettes highlight a fundamental fact about the psychotherapeutic craft, which makes mental health information and misinformation so difficult to navigate. Both of these people *benefited* from therapy, but—in my opinion—only one of them really *needed* it.

It's important to note that some therapists would disagree with me. These practitioners think everyone needs therapy. It's also important to note that therapists are financially incentivized to believe that absolutely everyone requires the services that therapists charge to provide. And yet, many other therapists agree with me, though some will never make such a declaration out loud because they would never want to risk inadvertently discouraging someone from seeking out therapy who actually really does need it. Even as I write these words, I share that concern.

The debate goes much deeper than whether or not we encourage treatment-seeking behavior. Some psychotherapists think that psychological problems are best described as illnesses, which reflects a perspective rooted in the medicalization of everyday life. Other practitioners support the notion that psychological problems are too broad and common to be described as illnesses. Some therapists believe that it is very rare for someone to genuinely have a mental disorder, and these therapists avoid diagnostic labels when they can. For these clinicians, people need help with "problems of living," not "illnesses." These therapists believe that what we call diagnoses are often normal responses to life's hardships and point out that therapy can be helpful for those who do not meet any diagnostic criteria. While many people might lean toward one side of the debate or the other, that does not mean that one side has more merit than the other.

I believe that both of these perspectives have value. Mental illness is real. I know because I've treated a lot of it. On the other hand, I understand that anxiety, depression, OCD, post-traumatic stress disorder (PTSD), and other mental illnesses are often normal responses to life's inevitable hardships. In other words, different people's nervous systems may manifest what we call diagnoses. If you lose your job and go broke, it's normal to feel depressed or anxious. Whether or not you need therapy to help you make sense of these feelings depends on a variety of factors, such as the severity of your symptoms and how long you deal with them.

Abby's and Bill's cases illustrate that different people need different approaches. For example, I was hesitant to label Abby with an anxiety disorder because, while she seemed nervous and self-conscious, her internal experience didn't really reflect a disturbance in her functioning. In other words, she did not meet the criteria for an anxiety diagnosis. Her treatment didn't require that I medicalize her experience. On the other hand, Bill's case required diagnostic language because he was already on medication for previously assigned diagnoses. A big part of his treatment was reassessing these labels and finding the correct ones. (As I explore in a later chapter, that's the thing about diagnosing: When done correctly, it can be a huge relief.)

When people insist that everyone needs therapy, I worry whether that sentiment redirects mental health resources from those who really need them (like Bill) to those with socioeconomic means to pay top dollar for the best therapist they can find. There is nothing immoral or unethical about taking advantage of therapy even if you don't technically need it. But it is also true that we may not have enough clinicians to treat everyone, which is increasingly making mental health care accessible only to a privileged few. If there is a limited supply, should the available resources go to the wealthy? What does it say about our culture and about how we approach life if the only way to solve problems of living is to speak to a trained professional? Can't we use other resources, such as coaches, for much of what we face? Can't we expect a certain level of support from our loved ones?

If you're trying to figure out whether you *need* to be in therapy, the best approach is to talk to a qualified professional. You can ask them how they define what a mental illness is and what it means for someone to not need to be in therapy. You should not let the idea that you might not need therapy stop you from going, and you should recognize that many people who need therapy resist going because of fear of what they may learn about themselves.

> **3 THINGS TO REMEMBER ABOUT MYTH #1: "EVERYONE SHOULD GO TO THERAPY"**
>
> 1. While anybody can *benefit* from therapy, not everyone *needs* therapy.
>
> 2. Therapy can help with problems of living, but it can also help with what we call mental disorders.
>
> 3. Remember, there are other ways to get help with life's problems.

Myth #2: "Analyzing Your Thoughts Is Always Good for You"

When Cara came to see me, it was clear she had been to therapy before. She already knew all the lingo. She appeared to be excellent at naming her feelings. She had a well-articulated understanding of how her childhood had impacted her as an adult. She could expatiate about her inner world for twenty minutes straight if I didn't interject some words of my own. Despite this awareness, she was still relatively low-functioning. She had a hard time keeping a job. She was living with extended family—reliant on their care—not because she wanted to be, but because she needed to be. She cried all the time and had a tough time in all types of relationships—with friends, coworkers, lovers, and others. She had been in therapy for years before seeing me. From what I could tell, her previous practitioner had mostly used an analytical approach. This therapist helped her uncover several repressed memories about the different traumas of her childhood, events she had no knowledge about prior to therapy.

Cara was a very different patient from Daniel. When Daniel came to see me, he was very reluctant to tell me what was going on. He wanted to be very clear about the rules concerning mandatory reporting, which typically involve instances when a therapist needs to break confidentiality because someone is at risk of hurting themselves or someone else. I initially thought he was potentially suicidal, but after a few sessions, he opened up to me. He was raised by a chef, and while he didn't work in the food industry, he loved cooking for his family, and it was a way he demonstrated his affection. Recently, he was dealing with disturbing thoughts. He told me about a night he was chopping vegetables and had a horrifying thought: "What if I used this knife to slice open one of my children?" Daniel was mortified. When I asked him what it was like to entertain these thoughts as actions he might carry out, he swore up and down that he would never ever hurt anyone, let alone his kids. Nevertheless, he was sick to his stomach that he could have such thoughts.

The idea that your thoughts mean something is a Freudian idea. Sigmund Freud—known as the father of psychoanalysis—understood your mind as an interplay between your consciousness and your subconscious. Simply put, your conscious mind is everything you are aware of, while your subconscious is everything outside of your awareness. Your mind builds defense mechanisms, sometimes called defense processes, to shield your conscious mind from painful material in your subconscious. This material could consist of emotions, beliefs, memories, carnal instincts, or anything else that we prefer to keep outside of our awareness. In traditional psychoanalysis, the therapist helps the patient become conscious of things they have pushed into their subconscious. When they become aware of these things, they should experience symptom relief.

Consider the case of Cara. She had been through quite a bit of psychoanalysis, but she hadn't gotten better and still wasn't getting better. In fact, her "recovered memories" seemed to be actively causing her distress. Now consider the case of Daniel. If you were his therapist, would you explore what these thoughts about his kitchen knife might have to do with potential subconscious material? Would it be therapeutic for him to consider that he might secretly have a deep unconscious desire to harm his own children, even though entertaining that idea filled him with shame and disgust? It's worth noting that the topic of repressed memories is a controversial one in the mental health field. Some find their existence to be self-evident, while others find the evidence to be sorely lacking.

There is more than one way to think about the mind. Freud's conception of the mind is not the only one. In the 1960s, another psychotherapist, Aaron Beck, came along. He noticed that traditional psychoanalysis was not making his patients better. He began to entertain the idea that maybe not all thoughts come from a deeper place. Maybe instead of analyzing thoughts to see whether they involved potential unconscious material, patients could learn how to criticize their thoughts. Beck coined the term *automatic cognitions*, which basically conveys the idea that sometimes thoughts are completely random. Other times, they are persistent and negative and come from illogical beliefs. According to Beck, thinking about your thoughts can lead to symptom relief because, often, patients will then start to think about their thoughts more clearly.

In the case of Daniel, I consulted with some colleagues, and we were able to assess that he did not present a danger to his children or anyone else. I proceeded to educate him that sometimes thoughts—even terrible ones—were totally random. They did not mean anything deeper. Therapists often call these "intrusive thoughts." For example, one common intrusive thought that people have is they are terrified they could be a pedophile. Having this thought does not mean that a person is attracted to minors. Everyone has random thoughts all the time, ranging from negative to amusing, from bizarre to commonplace. This does not mean that everyone has thoughts that cause them distress, which would require therapeutic attention. The trick is to understand which thoughts are worth diving more deeply into. Had I taken a more analytical approach with Daniel, I am not sure it would have been therapeutic.

In the case of Cara, she had spent considerable time analyzing her thoughts and exploring material in her subconscious, but she wasn't improving. In fact, according to her accounts of her previous therapy, it seemed that her symptoms had worsened with therapy. Instead of conducting more analysis with Cara, I suggested that we stop exploring her past. I offered that she had gained great insight into how her past affected her present, but we could use that insight to get better. We could practice different skills and consider navigating life differently from the way she had been living in recent years. We figured out what made sense based on her articulated counseling goals. With time, she began to recondition herself with tools we borrowed from behavioral therapy.

The behaviorists are really interesting thinkers because, unlike the analysts and the cognitive theorists, they almost don't care what you think or how you feel. Their priority is your behavior and how to help you recondition yourself to different patterns of behavior. For example, in Cara's case, she would often get overwhelmed trying new things. Her analysis was cogent—growing up, her parents ridiculed her for completing tasks appropriately. This is a particularly insidious form of emotional abuse. When people punish you for making a mistake, at least their response makes sense. In Cara's case, she would sometimes be punished for making mistakes but would sometimes also be punished for excelling at new things on her first try. Understandably, this unpredictability caused massive anxiety—even panic—when she tried something new. Learning to desensitize herself to her overwhelming feelings when she tried new things was a slow process. Over time, she became comfortable with it. Sometimes old triggers would come up when she encountered a novel situation, but together we were able to help desensitize her to the emotional overwhelm she experienced when trying new things.

Let me be clear: I am not saying that psychoanalysis isn't ever helpful. For one thing, I was trained analytically and regularly practiced what's called psychodynamic psychotherapy (essentially modern-day psychoanalysis). But I am not loyal to any single modality. In my practice, I like to do what works for the person in front of me. Sometimes you need to analyze. Sometimes you need to think about your thoughts. Other times you need to recondition yourself. Above all, remember that it's never a one-size-fits-all approach. Be cautious of advice that implies everything you think is significant. It's not, and we should be thankful for that fact.

**3 THINGS TO REMEMBER ABOUT MYTH #2:
"ANALYZING YOUR THOUGHTS IS
ALWAYS GOOD FOR YOU"**

1. Sometimes it's helpful to examine deeper meanings and subconscious material, but other times you need to think about your thoughts.

2. Occasionally a certain therapeutic modality can outlive its usefulness. If you are feeling stuck in therapy, ask your therapist whether they would consider a different approach or whether you might need a new therapist.

3. Don't believe everything you think.

Myth #3: "Expressing Your Feelings Is Valid"

Pretty much any therapist will tell you that all feelings are valid. I agree, but the word *valid* is widely misunderstood and often taken out of context. This contributes to a lot of confusion among mental health professionals and patients alike. For example, by *valid*, do we mean "having a sound basis in logic or fact" or "reasonable and cogent"? Anyone who has ever dealt with an emotionally difficult situation can tell you that definition does not apply. Emotions, even normative and pleasant ones, are not always logical and reasonable.

Therapists are often *validating* feelings and emotions their patients experience. What does this mean? By validating feelings, therapists are declaring that the feelings being discussed are understandable and worthy of consideration. It's okay to feel them. In fact, when it comes to your mental health, it's often necessary. That is not the same thing as saying that all feelings are reasonable or all feelings are worth acting on. It's certainly not the same thing as saying that all feelings are rational or even helpful. Yet therapists, myself included, continue to validate our patients anyway. Why? Therapists are so obsessed with validating feelings because many mental health symptoms are correlated with emotional suppression.

Whenever I think about emotional suppression, I think of my patient Elizabeth. Elizabeth was happily married with three children. She didn't love her job but said it was good enough. Her marriage wasn't perfect, but she loved her partner. Her kids were not without challenges, but overall she loved being a mom. So why was she feeling so stressed and anxious all the time? It was apparent to me from our first session together that Elizabeth spent a lot of energy in her own head. She was a highly rational person. Elizabeth was a textbook intellectualizer, meaning she used thinking to avoid feeling. Anyone can be thoughtful, cerebral, rational, or logical without intellectualizing. I could tell that Elizabeth was intellectualizing because the intellectualization accompanied her anxiety. Instead of saying that she felt annoyed when her teenager talked back to her, she would go on scattered tangents about the situation without naming that she felt annoyed. When her boss asked her to stay late, she didn't report feeling anything, but she did elaborate on the reasons her boss depended on her more than on her colleagues.

In some ways, Elizabeth's treatment was very straightforward. I spent a lot of time reflecting and validating her emotions. I helped her practice getting out of her head and feeling her emotions in her body. Therapists have people focus on the bodily sensation of an emotion because it's often a way to let the emotion get fully processed. As she practiced doing this, her levels of anxiety went down. It's important to note that there can be other etiologies, otherwise known as origins or root causes, of anxiety symptoms besides emotional suppression. It's not uncommon for the first therapeutic intervention to not totally do the trick. In this case, I had nailed it the first time. I didn't treat Elizabeth for very long before she got what she needed and I sent her on her merry way.

For a patient like Elizabeth, validating feelings is central to the therapy process. One way I like to talk to patients about their feelings is to articulate that their feelings are data and their body and brain are the processing system. You can interpret data any number of ways. For example, Elizabeth learned that it was okay to share that she was feeling frustrated or annoyed when her family demanded too much of her. She communicated this in a responsible and respectful way. Other times, it was better not to share her feelings. For example, one time a coworker made a mistake that caused Elizabeth extra work. She got angry. But it wouldn't have been helpful for Elizabeth to yell at her coworker (even though that might have felt good). Instead, she felt her emotion, chose not to act on it, and proceeded differently.

Not every patient needs to feel their feelings deeply to get better. I am reminded of Frankie, a patient of mine who showed up to his first appointment visibly upset and crying, and then shared that he actually went to the wrong office in the building and felt really rejected when the receptionist didn't have an appointment for him. Does it make sense to feel unpleasant things when you find yourself in the wrong place? Of course. Does that mean it's mentally healthy to express anger at the receptionist of a dentist office when you're looking for a behavioral health clinic? I would argue no, it's not. Treatment with Frankie did not look like spending lots of time feeling his feelings and being in his body. It was about learning to tolerate overwhelming emotions without acting on them. He actually benefited from learning to think instead of feel. One could argue that he learned to intellectualize more and feel his feelings less.

That's the thing about defense processes such as intellectualizing: From a psychoanalytic perspective, they help you avoid unpleasant unconscious material, including unpleasant feelings. Defenses are not good or bad—just as feelings are not good or bad (notice how I like to describe them as pleasant or unpleasant). Whether referring to a feeling or a defense, it all depends on how they are used.

I'll end by telling you a personal story. Once I was dating someone, and we really hit it off quickly. One day, I noticed the person had turned read receipts on for their text messages and had left mine on read. Believe me, I had feelings about this. But I didn't express them to this person. I didn't suppress them either. It's understandable that being left on read can make you feel ignored and not like a priority. In my head, I was so suspicious: *Are they talking to lots of other love interests? Are they already bored of me? Are they playing mind games with me?* (See the previous chapter about not listening to all your thoughts.) It took some effort to reel in that inner dialogue before I could come up with other ways to interpret the read receipts.

In the end, I brought the topic up the next time I saw the person. As it turns out, they had actually gotten the new iPhone that day and didn't realize their read receipts were turned on. If I had expressed my feelings or let my internal monologue run wild, I could have ended up starting a dialogue with the person that was less than reasonable. I could have texted them about it, sure. But that's not how I interpreted my emotions at that time.

So the next time you think about your feelings, consider

whether or not it's better to feel them. Consider whether or not it's helpful for you to act on them. And remember that the only people who get to express and act on every emotion they have the second they have them are children. When we raise our children, we teach them how to be in better control of their emotions. This is not the same thing as invalidating whatever their emotions happen to be.

> **3 THINGS TO REMEMBER ABOUT MYTH #3: "EXPRESSING YOUR FEELINGS IS VALID"**
>
> 1. Validating feelings in a therapeutic context is different from validating them in a nontherapeutic context.
>
> 2. Feelings are data points, and you can choose to interpret them any way you want to.
>
> 3. You don't need to act on every emotion you feel.

Myth #4: "You Were Totally Projecting When That Happened"

Have you heard of John Smid? He once ran a gay conversion camp. Decades later, he accepted himself as a homosexual and came out. I don't bring this story up to judge him. Yes, it's unfortunate that it took him a long time to accept himself. No, I don't approve of the fact that he psychologically harmed many people along the way. Isn't it curious, though? Isn't it interesting to consider what was going on with his psyche to live his life that way—conducting himself in a way that was contrary to who he was and how he felt deep down?

Everyone loves to conduct armchair psychoanalysis. Folks constantly observe one another's behavior and guess at deeper motivations, even if they are not therapists. We do this with our loved ones, in business, and on dates. As psychological terms become more mainstream, people often use and misuse the same tired popular terms to conduct their analyses. The danger is that they can miss the mark. For example, when I saw *Boy Erased* (a movie that depicts John Smid as a conversion program leader), I heard many people exclaim that he must have been *projecting*.

A person who represses their sexuality and spends a lifetime and a career trying to eradicate it from the world is not exactly projecting. Projection is just one of many defense mechanisms, which are sometimes called defense processes. In Smid's case, I would guess that he was engaging in something called reaction formation. Reaction formation occurs when people express the opposite of what they truly feel, sometimes to an exaggerated extent, because they deem what they feel to be unacceptable for some reason. Smid's reaction formation manifested as efforts to change other people's homosexuality, because he found it unacceptable that he could not truly change himself. If John were projecting, he would have assumed that many people he met were actually closeted gay people, even if they were not actually gay. Projection happens when unwanted thoughts, feelings, or motivations are readily seen in others—they appear as threats from outside yourself. For example, it's common for people who are uncomfortable with their own anger to accuse others of having hostile motivations.

Now I would like to explain how psychoanalysis works so you can better conduct your own armchair analysis. When I learned about psychoanalysis in grad school, I had a professor discourage us from asking *why* questions. Instead, he encouraged us to ask *how* questions. Instead of asking someone why they became a stockbroker, ask them how they became a stockbroker. Asking someone a why-driven question assumes that they know why they are doing something, but anyone who studies the human mind is aware that this is rarely the case. If we asked John Smid why he became a conversion camp leader, chances are he would not have been able to articulate his repressed homosexuality. If you asked him how he became a conversion camp leader, however, he might have responded with clues from his past that revealed his deeper motivations.

That's the first lesson I want you to remember when you try to analyze others: They may not be conscious of the thing that you are suspicious of, so don't expect them to be more aware than they are. Many people get into all sorts of interpersonal drama when they expect or insist that others see things the way that they themselves see things. This is a waste of time. Don't get curious about *why*; get curious about *how*. This brings me to my second point.

An old aphorism suggests that "the smartest people realize they know very little, because it takes a lot of knowledge to understand the scope of your own ignorance." It's derived from the Dunning–Kruger effect, which occurs when a person's lack of knowledge allows them to overestimate their own competence. It makes sense. People who do not know enough about a subject don't have the knowledge to identify the mistakes that arise from gaps in their knowledge. The same is true about self-awareness. Don't fool yourself into thinking that you are free from your own biases. As the person trying to conduct the analysis, you are limited by your own experience and knowledge and by your own psyche's defenses. The most self-aware people I know are people who understand they still have a lot to learn about themselves.

If you want to analyze with more sophistication, you can't assume that you can view a person in your life objectively. There's no way around this. Proper psychoanalysis requires an objective practitioner who has no outside relationship to the patient—but even an objective practitioner has biases. Instead of analyzing people as if you don't have any biases, you can actually use your biases to your advantage. In order to understand how this works, you also need to understand something called transference.

Old-school psychoanalysis is often depicted with the patient lying on a couch looking at the ceiling. There is no eye contact with the therapist. One of the reasons for this practice is that the psychoanalyst is trying to be a blank slate. The idea is that, over time, the patient will begin having thoughts and feelings about the therapist. These thoughts and feelings are examples of transference and are clues to the dynamics of the patient's subconscious. Here's the thing: In order for a therapist to properly conduct this sort of therapy, they have to be aware of their countertransference. *Countertransference* is the term for the thoughts and feelings therapists have about their patients and can be clues into the ways their own unconscious processes are playing a role in the therapeutic dynamic. It can be tricky to learn what is countertransference and what is an acceptable interpretation of the person you are trying to analyze.

My patient Gabriella was twenty-one years old and living with her parents; she told me stories of abuse that conjured a visceral sense of wanting to protect her and get her out of that house. The impulse to rescue her was tied to the thought that she was not able to get out herself. Was that a cogent understanding of her situation? Did it have to do with some unconscious desire I have to rescue or fix people? Or was my countertransference a clue—an insight—into how her family and others in her life viewed her?

One of the ways Gabriella's family was cruel to her was in their eagerness to remind her that she wasn't good enough to live on her own. If I leaned into my impulse to try to give her all the help and advice she needed, I risked re-creating a dynamic that plagued many of her familial relationships. I would have been another person in her life who believed she couldn't do the things she wanted to do for herself. I share this story because I want to be clear that having countertransference does not make me or anyone a bad therapist. As I said, you can use it to conduct a more "objective" analysis of the situation. Countertransference can be used to support the therapeutic relationship, even if the countertransference had nothing to do with my personal unconscious dynamics. That's important to note: Just because it's countertransference, that doesn't mean it's inaccurate or unhelpful.

When conducting an analysis, it's important to consider what your goal is with the person. When I analyze in a professional setting, it's always to help the person in front of me gain deeper self-awareness on a relevant issue. Many people complain that therapy consists of continuously talking about why they are the way they are, without anything changing. That's why I am not a purist when it comes to the analytical approach. Other types of therapy may be needed to help these individuals with their goals.

I would leave you with the same advice. Consider the function of your desire to analyze someone else. Is it so you can get along better? Is it so you can get something you want from the other person? More often than not, I find that when someone is constantly analyzing another's behavior, they already have the insight they need. They just need to put the insight to use—or accept that they simply like to pontificate about it.

3 THINGS TO REMEMBER ABOUT MYTH #4: "YOU WERE TOTALLY PROJECTING WHEN THAT HAPPENED"

1. Everyone armchair-analyzes.

2. It's better to get curious about *how* rather than about *why*. The latter inquiry often involves too much bias when it comes to you or the subject of your analysis.

3. Biases are going to come up when you analyze people, so lean into them. Don't be in denial about them.

Myth #5: "Personality Frameworks Are Reductive, Inaccurate, and Not Helpful"

Myers-Briggs. Enneagram. Human Design. Five-Factor Model. StrengthsFinder. Astrology. Personality tests seem to be everywhere. Whether the test is evidence-based or spiritual, if it's some sort of typing system, I was probably obsessed with it during some phase of my life. If you're someone who loves personality frameworks—or if you know someone who does—then you are aware that people who love these things can be very enthusiastic about sharing the framework with others. They want people in their life to take the quiz, learn the framework, and talk to them about it.

What if I told you that personality frameworks don't need to be scientific or accurate in order to be helpful? What if I told you that people who think that personality frameworks are too reductive to be useful are completely missing the point? What would your reaction be? By the end of this chapter, not only will you understand what I mean, but you will also be armed with knowledge to navigate the world of personality frameworks and psychometric testing. Personality frameworks are systems used to organize someone's personality. By *personality*, we mean someone's pervasive patterns of thinking, feeling, and behaving. Psychometrics is a field dedicated to measuring, assessing, testing, and diagnosing various psychological phenomena. Whether you're seeing a psychologist for a formal testing battery or your date wants to know whether you two are compatible, this chapter is full of stuff you *need* to know.

Many people do not like personality typing systems because they think they are supposed to be super accurate, like a blood test. For example, many will criticize Myers-Briggs for not being evidence-based. Others will criticize the Five-Factor Model, which is evidence-based. Ironically, the Five-Factor Model was constructed over decades by psychologists collaborating across different countries and cultures all over the world. The literature is very strong. Even when these typing systems are rigorously studied and designed, people often criticize them by saying something like "human beings are more complicated than that." Critics point to the limited nature of the framework in question. These resources get an unfair reputation. If you understand how they work, that knowledge will help you to differentiate scientific and unscientific psychological frameworks and to identify which unscientific ones are still enormously helpful.

First, let's distinguish between frameworks and tests. By *tests*, I mean proper psychometric tools that measure something about your psychology. Frameworks may have a test you can take to figure out which *type* you are, as the Enneagram does. At the same time, you can still learn about the Enneagram framework without ever taking a test. Conversely, some tests measure psychological phenomena that are not attached to a framework. For example, the Patient Health Questionnaire-9, or PHQ-9, is a test that you might take at your doctor's office during a yearly checkup. The test measures to what extent you are experiencing symptoms of depression. Depression, as it's defined, is not exactly the type of framework that attempts to organize personality. And plenty of studies, writings, and philosophies on the subject of personality don't accompany a framework at all.

Whether or not a test happens to be accurate likely depends on how the test is designed. This discussion takes us a bit into the weeds, but it's information that's important to know if you want to be a pro at navigating personality tests. If designed properly, a test measures traits that are *valid* and *reliable*. *Validity* is about how accurate a test is at measuring what it says it will measure, in the sense that an arrow hits the target it's aiming for. For a test to be truly accurate, that arrow must also hit the target consistently. That's why tests also need to be *reliable*. *Reliability* refers to the extent to which a test is consistent. A test needs to be both valid and reliable in order to be truly accurate. Think about it: If a test is valid but not reliable, then it's not very accurate. If a test is reliable but measures something different from what it purports to measure—well, that is not accurate either.

In psychology, accurately measuring personality is tricky. That trickiness ends up giving personality frameworks a bad rap. People get lost in the conversation about validity, reliability, accuracy, and applicability but forget the most important thing: Personality frameworks are reductive by design. In fact, personality as a concept is reductive by design! A personality trait points to a pattern that transcends context, but that does not mean that a personality trait is rigid. For example, it's normal for a true extrovert to need alone time sometimes, but they're correctly identified as an extrovert if they are generally enthusiastic, assertive, and gregarious.

While it's true that different tests vary in accuracy, the most important thing about a personality framework is not the accuracy of the test. It's about using the framework as a lens to deepen your understanding. When we reduce the complexity of a human being down to a framework, we can illuminate something new about them and talk about that part of them with more specificity. It's about being able to more effectively connect and communicate with one another.

Here's how that works: In a series of academic papers called "Rhetoric Lobotomized," Professor Dave Logan, of the University of Southern California, introduced the idea of *terministic screens*. Over time, while learning a new subject, you develop a jargon. For example, when I went to school to become a therapist, I learned a lot of new words and distinctions about psychology. After a while, once you have sufficiently mastered enough words, you have an aha moment: Everything clicks and you see the world in a new way. You experience deep understanding. You see things through a terministic screen—a lens you gained by learning words. Now everything you see is colored by this new lens, and no matter what you do, someone who has not done the work to have that lens cannot see what you see. This is the reason doctors speak in layman's terms to their patients, and lawyers simplify case law for their clients. It's the reason that, when I speak to someone during a session, I do *not* say things like "Your maladaptive coping mechanisms exacerbate symptomatology." I say: "If you continue to overschedule yourself, you will continue to feel overwhelmed."

Personality frameworks are like terministic screens. For example, the book *The Five Love Languages,* by Gary Chapman, is a tool designed to help couples better communicate how to give and receive affection.[1] Many people learn the love languages and say something like "Well, I like all of those" or "I'm more than one." That's totally fine, but what matters is not whether the framework is scientifically accurate or not. For couples therapy, what matters is whether it helps the members of the couple see each other in a new way. My two cents is that it does not matter if Human Design is unscientific or informed by astrology. As long as it's being used to communicate more effectively, it has a practicality worth embracing.

So yes, personality typing systems and many psychological frameworks are reductive; that's the point. They allow us to access different ways to understand and communicate with one another.

3 THINGS TO REMEMBER ABOUT MYTH #5: "PERSONALITY FRAMEWORKS ARE REDUCTIVE, INACCURATE, AND NOT HELPFUL"

1. Personality frameworks don't need to be accurate or evidence-based to be helpful.

2. Personality frameworks are helpful because they are reductive, not in spite of their limited scope.

3. The promise of these frameworks is that they can help you see others differently and communicate with them in a more effective way.

Myth #6: "Hurt People Hurt People"

If you've been hurt by someone, and you have gained solace from understanding their motivations as coming from their own pain, then I need you to know that this chapter might not be for you. This chapter deconstructs the idea that "hurt people hurt people" by holding it up to scrutiny. While I believe that this saying is more of a myth than an aphorism, I acknowledge that it can be true in some cases. Even though the saying does give comfort to many people, it can also be used as an excuse to justify ongoing abuse and mistreatment. This idea is sometimes used by those suffering from ongoing abuse as a rationale to remain in unhealthy, and potentially dangerous, situations. Most insidiously, this idea is also sometimes used as a way to justify hurting others. For that reason, I feel I must hold this myth up to scrutiny.

When thinking about the myth "hurt people hurt people," I am reminded of my patient Hugh, who grew up in a physically and verbally abusive home. He was the middle child of several brothers. Their parents would regularly hit them for punishment. After he left home, he reported never getting into a fight again. We can't even say that he emotionally hurt others due to a trauma response. Hugh was, in many ways, the epitome of masculinity. He was rugged, handsome, muscular, and stoic. Like many men, he didn't show much emotion, but unlike many men, he didn't show much anger either. He was not violent or aggressive, but he was still very strong in demeanor. I remember always being specifically impressed by these qualities. His composure was a maintaining factor in his mental illness. His anger was so repressed that he never really said a harsh thing to anyone. This repression manifested in serious depressive symptoms, which ultimately brought him in to see me. It's not accurate to say that he opened up to me and then experienced symptom relief. It's more accurate to say that he opened up to himself, felt his feelings, and then experienced healing. I can't recall a time he ever showed any emotional hostility toward me. Even with all his ruggedness and strength, he was one of the more subdued individuals I ever got to know.

The truth is, human beings respond to difficult situations in a wide variety of ways. Like Hugh, many people who have been hurt are exceedingly cautious about accidentally hurting others. Some survivors end up hurting themselves, either through direct self-harm or in more indirect ways such as living recklessly or self-sabotaging. I am not sure whether "hurt people hurt people" applies if the person being hurt is themselves. Furthermore, the saying is simply not logical. If every single person who was hurt went on to hurt others, then we would all be abusers. No one experiences life without being hurt. Therefore, the idea that all hurt people hurt people doesn't make that much logical or mathematical sense.

When it comes to people who *do* hurt people, I want to point out several different kinds of abusers. One kind consists of people who are psychologically immature. Young children often get into tiffs with one another, as you can readily see at your nearest day care. Most of us get socialized out of this behavior, but some people struggle with it into adulthood. I would not argue that people who hurt others out of a developmental delay have necessarily been hurt. It's important to note that I am not referring to people with a diagnosable developmental disability. Lots of people develop certain capacities at different rates than others, and that is quite normal. Of course, many children with clinically significant social and behavioral issues have been hurt, and I do not want to discount their experiences. But many young children who push and shove need to be socialized properly, or they risk perpetrating hurt from a place of psychological immaturity. Many adults do the same, often emotionally, from a place of psychological immaturity.

Another group of people who hurt others are people who lash out when they are emotionally dysregulated. These individuals are like balloons; they get filled with pressure until one day they explode. They may not even remember the explosion afterward. Some people report "seeing red" and can even be dismayed with themselves when they realize what they have done. Emotional dysregulation *can* be a symptom of being hurt in your past, but there are lots of reasons people may have a hard time regulating emotions such as anger. *Hypomania* is the term used when people who have bipolar disorder go through periods of sleeplessness and high energy. In hypomania, people can be super elated. At other times, hypomania can lead people to feel extremely agitated and lash out. Withdrawal from substances can lead to abusive behavior, too.

A third group of people are more calculating in how they go about hurting others. These people likely have lower levels of empathy. They don't "see red," and they are not acting out because their emotions are heightened. My suspicion is that the person who gets dysregulated and "sees red" before hurting someone is more likely to have been hurt themselves, although I cannot find any literature supporting this claim. Their previous experiences may contribute to difficulty regulating their emotions. But some people's heart rates do not rise when they strike other people. Some people remain cool as a cucumber. You have to wonder whether that sort of person was hurt or is simply wired differently. It's worth noting that not everyone with deficits in empathy is a psychopath. The fact remains that hurting someone because of a lower capacity for empathy is not the same thing as hurting someone because of a past hurt.

I am also not totally clear on how the saying "hurt people hurt people" applies to emotional hurt. Emotional hurt is deeply subjective. For example, an off-color joke may hurt someone's feelings, but it could bring someone else laughter and joy. With physical hurt, the perpetrator and victim are more often obvious. With emotional hurt, there is an element of subjectivity that may not always render the perpetrator intentional or guilty. For example, would a vulnerable narcissist, someone who goes out of their way to play the victim card, be given the same leeway to claim they have been emotionally hurt as anyone else?

Given the subjectivity of emotional hurt, the idea that "emotionally hurt people emotionally hurt people" only deepens confusion and renders the saying even more unhelpful and unclear. Distinguishing emotional abuse from the experience of typical emotional pain offers yet another example of how therapy-speak can make things more confusing than clear. I am particularly fond of the way therapist and life coach Logan Cohen defines emotional abuse. He describes emotional abuse as an act that is meant to cause shame, guilt, fear, or some other unpleasant emotion. In that moment of disorientation, the abuser has an opportunity to control their subject. In a conversation with Logan, I asked him whether he thought it "counted" as emotional abuse if the act was unintentional or if it was coming from a place of hurt. According to Logan, that doesn't matter, because the impact is still the same. He told me that one can have compassion for people who act from a place of woundedness without justifying or rationalizing their behavior. I couldn't agree more.

---

3 THINGS TO REMEMBER ABOUT MYTH #6: "HURT PEOPLE HURT PEOPLE"

1. Some hurt people hurt people, but many hurt people go out of their way to never hurt anyone, physically or emotionally.

2. Many people who survive difficult experiences hurt themselves, directly or indirectly.

3. There are many reasons why people who do hurt others take those actions.

Part II

DSM Mayhem: Common Myths About Mental Health Diagnoses

Myth #7: "Receiving a Diagnosis Is Terrible"

When people go to therapy, it's a common fear that they will receive a diagnosis. When I ask people—patients or peers—why getting a diagnosis makes them nervous, they often report wanting to avoid being besmirched by a label. In other words, people think that receiving a diagnosis means they're crazy. In actuality, receiving a mental health diagnosis is often a good thing, assuming the diagnosis is accurate. A diagnosis is simply one clinician's opinion of how you might be helped. In fact, being properly labeled is typically a relief to those who receive a diagnosis. One of the main reasons clinicians diagnose is to inform a treatment plan. For example, the reason there's a difference between the diagnosis of ADHD and the diagnosis of Bipolar II is that treatment is meaningfully different, even though the two conditions can look somewhat similar.

Isabel was initially scared of getting a diagnosis. When she came to see me, she was transferring to another college and hoping that therapy would help her get a fresh start. I remember her getting quite emotional telling me the story of her life. She said she felt "insane" because she got so much more emotional than everyone else. Isabel described intense abandonment issues that only seemed to be getting worse, because the more she acted emotionally, the more friends seemed to back away. She was hopeful that she could find a sense of who she was with therapy, but she was scared that I would label her with something bad.

Receiving a diagnosis is not the worst thing that can happen to you in therapy. There are two other things that can happen to you that are even worse. One is that you can receive an incorrect diagnosis. Because diagnoses inform treatment plans, a misdiagnosis can result in a treatment that doesn't work. For example, someone who is experiencing insomnia due to undiagnosed OCD is going to receive a completely different type of treatment from someone diagnosed with Bipolar II. The way you work with disordered behavior—including disordered sleep—in OCD is wildly different from treatment in bipolar spectrum disorders. This issue initially made Isabel quite anxious. Now she had two fears: fear of getting diagnosed and being officially labeled as crazy and fear of getting diagnosed incorrectly and having therapy not work.

I explained to Isabel that sometimes people are so complex that nobody can quite describe what is going on with them in terms of their mental health. This is the other thing that can happen to you in therapy, which is, in my opinion, worse than receiving a diagnosis. When we can't name what we're seeing, mental health professionals don't always know how to help. Think about it: If we can't name it, then we can't read a book about it, do research, or even discuss it with colleagues with any sort of efficiency. One nice thing about diagnostic language is that it gives clinicians a shorthand to use in communicating with one another. For example, when I say "major depressive disorder" to another clinician, they have a pretty good idea of what I mean. Using that term is way more expedient than reciting a long list of symptoms would be.

Here is something I did not explain to Isabel, but that I want to explain to you because it's worth knowing. Sometimes, when a patient is highly complex and people can't quite describe what is happening with them, they receive multiple diagnoses. While some people certainly do meet the criteria of multiple diagnoses, it's my opinion that many people who receive multiple diagnoses don't actually meet those criteria. It seems to me that their previous clinician didn't know what was wrong with them, so they just threw the kitchen sink at them. The reason I push back against this tendency is that, often, multiple diagnoses don't really inform us about how to help the person. The one exception might be with respect to medication. The way psychiatrists diagnose to justify a prescription is different from your typical psychotherapist, but the idea is still the same. You decide on the label to determine a treatment plan—only with a psychiatrist, it's about prescribing medication.

I told Isabel that since she was paying me out of pocket (I didn't accept insurance at that time), I didn't need to diagnose her with anything; I would diagnose her if it was accurate and would be helpful for her case. I also explained that if she really wanted to be sure that the diagnosis was accurate, we could send her to a diagnostician—a psychologist who specializes in psychological assessment and testing. All clinicians are trained to diagnose, but not all clinicians specialize in psychological testing. The nice thing about psychological testing is that you don't just receive a diagnosis. You get a whole report full of subjective and objective data that your therapist can use to inform a treatment plan. It's not always useful for your therapist to take this approach. They can if they're trained in it. Plenty of shrinks who are trained in psychological testing will bring their patients through a testing battery.

I find it helpful to get an objective pair of eyes if a proper diagnosis is warranted. In my practice, I occasionally refer patients to testing psychologists, and patients always find it helpful and worthwhile. This was the case with Isabel. After a few days of testing with the psychologist, Isabel learned that she almost met the criteria for borderline personality disorder. While she had a lot of the symptoms, she didn't check enough boxes. Isabel and I looked at the report together. She initially felt a lot of shame about having something like a personality disorder. She also felt anxious about not meeting the full criteria because she thought that it meant I didn't know how to help her.

That's when I explained to her that we could still use the research and practices that guide treatment for borderline personality disorder. In fact, because she didn't meet the full criteria, it was arguable that treatment was more likely to be successful. Research shows that people who remain in treatment for borderline personality disorder can get better and enter remission.[1] Essentially, her prognosis—the likely outcome of her diagnosis—was promising because she had fewer symptoms than the full diagnosis required. An important sidenote: Every section of the Diagnostic and Statistical Manual of Mental Disorders, Fifth Edition (DSM-V), has criteria for people who fit some diagnostic criteria but not all of them.

Isabel's case was a successful one. She got a diagnosis, even though it didn't fit the neat boundaries of diagnostic categories. She remained committed to treatment. Dialectical behavior therapy is one way you work with borderline personality disorder. I combined that approach with something called intersubjective psychotherapy, a form of psychodynamic therapy in which the practitioner brings a lot of themselves into the room and helps the patient figure things out from a highly collaborative perspective. After a while, Isabel accomplished her counseling goals. She had better control over her behaviors and emotions. She had the skills to deal with distressing thoughts. She felt she could maintain long-term relationships with friends and romantic partners. As far as Isabel and I were concerned, getting a diagnosis was a success.

If you are considering therapy or are discussing diagnostic labels with your therapist, I hope you remember Isabel's story. We used diagnostic criteria as a tool to understand her, but her care team—her doctor, her testing psychologist, and myself—were not overly preoccupied with trying to determine what did or didn't constitute psychopathology. Diagnosis was just one of many things that happened to Isabel during her treatment. It was decidedly not the worst thing that could have happened to her.

> **3 THINGS TO REMEMBER ABOUT MYTH #7:**
> **"RECEIVING A DIAGNOSIS IS TERRIBLE"**
>
> 1. Being diagnosed is not the worst thing that can happen to you in therapy.
>
> 2. The worst thing that can happen to you in therapy is that no one is able to figure out what's wrong with you.
>
> 3. Proper diagnosis should be a relief, because it means the mental health field can help you.

⊗ Myth #8: "Mental Health Diagnoses Are Just Made-Up"

I am going to let you in on a piece of slang that typically only mental health professionals understand: *DSM-basher*. As we've seen, *DSM* stands for "Diagnostic and Statistical Manual of Mental Disorders" (*DSM-V* refers to the current fifth edition). I first encountered the amusing term *DSM-basher* when I read Dr. Robert McNally's book *What Is a Mental Illness?* McNally, a Harvard professor, writes "I am not a DSM-basher" as he criticizes his fellow clinicians for needlessly trashing diagnostic criteria and the DSM, sometimes referred to as the bible of psychiatry.[1]

A DSM-basher is a mental health clinician who unnecessarily criticizes the DSM but also the idea of diagnosis in general. Such a clinician will often say things like "The DSM is culturally insensitive and therefore inherently problematic" and "Most patients who walk into my office don't fit into the neat little boxes of the DSM criteria, so why bother?" It's true that there are cogent criticisms of the DSM on cultural grounds, but the DSM-V added something called a Cultural Formation Interview to address that criticism.[2] The Cultural Formation Interview was added to the DSM to help clinicians maintain the integrity of diagnostic categories, while gaining a better understanding of how nuanced cultural factors impact their patients. It's also true that individual experiences of mental illness don't always fit into neat diagnostic categories when people seek mental health treatment. But the DSM—while imperfect—is actually very important.

Diagnostic labels do not apply to every situation in which there is a mental health concern, but that does not mean that diagnostic criteria are simply "made-up." Diagnostic criteria are constructed by researchers and practitioners all over the world. Diagnostic labels—such as *anxiety, depression, trauma,* and so on—may change as the mental health field evolves, but that does not mean that diagnostic labels do not have value. Some people are critical of diagnostic criteria because the framework of diagnosis has limited utility. Unfortunately, some clinicians confuse limited utility with zero utility. By writing off the value of diagnostic criteria altogether, mental health professionals may be causing more problems than they are solving.

To understand why diagnoses are important, we need to consider the philosophy of categories. When we communicate to one another, we categorize things. We take things that exist on a continuum, and we break them down into simple and categorical groups. We do this to save time. We refer to simple schemas to get our point across more efficiently. For example, when we talk about color, we take the full range of all the colors that exist and break them down into the categories of red, orange, yellow, green, blue, indigo, and violet. To a certain extent, the boundaries we put in between these colors are arbitrary. At a paint store, for example, you can easily be overwhelmed by the sheer range of blue paints that are available. It is not convenient or useful for most of us to communicate by saying "cyan" or "cerulean" or "capri" or "cobalt" instead of "blue." Most of us are not artists or trying to sell different kinds of paint or design a cerulean belt. For most of us, it's too complicated to learn or remember or use all the different names for types of blue, so we settle for the broad category "blue" when we communicate.

Categories are used for different reasons. The first involves what are known as classical categories, which we use to determine how things are similar and how they are different. One example of a classical category is shape. A triangle has three sides and three angles, and the sum of the three angles always equals 180 degrees. If you don't have those three features, you are not a triangle. There is no exception to this rule. Another example is chemistry. If you have two hydrogen molecules and one oxygen molecule, then you get to be a water molecule. That is it. There are no ifs, ands, or buts to these classical categories.

Shapes and chemical molecules are categorized in the classical sense, but paint colors belong in family resemblance categories. The *Stanford Encyclopedia of Philosophy* states, "Family resemblance exhibits the lack of boundaries and the distance from exactness that characterize different uses of the same concept."[3] In other words, we don't just use categories to group things that have a single common defining feature, like molecules or shapes. We also use categories to group things that have similarities, such as colors and mental health diagnoses. In the DSM-V, the point of categorizing a patient with a diagnosis is so they can receive treatment. The category, label, or diagnosis is not classical because depression can look slightly different for everyone. Whether one person has a manifestation of depression that looks one way and someone else has a manifestation that looks another way, we call these things depression because—theoretically—the treatment for depression is similar nonetheless.

Consider the criteria for panic disorder. Thirteen different traits are a characteristic of a panic attack. Still, an individual needs to display only four of them to be having a panic attack. This implies that three people can have a panic attack with each one looking completely different. Why should we categorize panic attacks this way? Well, the reason is that psychiatrists, psychologists, and therapists are not scientists, not in the sense that a chemist who uses classical categories is a scientist. Therapists don't categorize symptomology the way a scientist might categorize triangles or molecules. Therapists are practitioners; they use categories not to make clean distinctions but to construct a proper treatment plan. The three individuals experiencing a panic attack may display different symptoms, but because their symptoms are in a family resemblance category known as panic disorder, the treatment protocol for all three individuals follows a similar goal—reducing symptoms and getting their panic attacks under control.

In research, categorizations are significant because we want to ensure that we are all discussing the same thing. This is called *construct validity,* meaning that what you're studying is the thing you think you're studying. For example, suppose different researchers in different universities want to study depression. In that case, it's helpful for the definition of major depressive disorder (MDD) to be consistent across the different labs and studies. In clinical practice, it's also beneficial to have consistent definitions across different settings. If I am treating a patient struggling with MDD and I reach out to a specialist, it's helpful to know we are discussing the same thing. I am not arguing that we should be overly rigid in our conceptualization of different mental health problems. I agree that it's important to think outside the box and not rely solely on diagnostic criteria. At the same time, the mental health culture needs to be aligned on what different terms mean. Whether in research, clinical case consultation, or the media, it's vital for definitions to be consistent, or we risk devolving further into psychobabble.

**3 THINGS TO REMEMBER ABOUT MYTH #8:
"MENTAL HEALTH DIAGNOSES ARE JUST MADE-UP"**

1. Diagnostic labels do not apply to every situation in which there is a mental health concern, but that does not mean that diagnostic criteria are simply made-up.

2. Construct validity of diagnoses matters for ongoing mental health practice and research.

3. Words have definitions, and diagnostic criteria are one way for mental health culture to stay aligned on different definitions.

⊗
Myth #9: "Your Diagnosis Is Your Identity"

In her stand-up comedy special *Look at You*, the comedian Taylor Tomlinson discloses to all her fans that she was diagnosed with bipolar disorder. When she learned her diagnosis, her provider told her something like "If it makes you feel better, you don't have to say, 'I *am* bipolar'—you can say, 'I *have* bipolar." Taylor shares her hilarious musings with the audience: "Which feels a lot like someone going, 'I said you were *being* a bitch'"—as opposed to saying that you *are* just a bitch.[1]

This bit is brilliant because so many therapists—myself included—are such sticklers about saying that diagnoses are things you *have*, not things you *are*. Taylor's joke does make me wonder whether these semantics do anything at all to help people accept their diagnoses or combat stigma in a meaningful way. While the difference may just be semantics, I do think it is an important one.

There are many reasons someone might look for a mental health diagnosis to explain who they are. I think this is the main one: Therapy can be a process in which you learn a lot about who you are as a person. In fact, identity development happens in therapy *all the time.* Therapy is also a process in which you may or may not receive a diagnosis. It makes sense to me that many people then mistakenly assume that a diagnosis says a lot about who you are as a person.

It's also very normal, when receiving a diagnosis, to notice how much it explains about you and your behavior, feelings, internal monologue, and so on. I really empathize with people who grab onto their diagnosis like a lifeboat in a storm. Diagnosis can be an incredibly valuable treatment tool. Diagnoses are made for treatment plans. If your treatment isn't working, it's possible the diagnosis is incorrect or your counseling goals are not adequately captured by a diagnostic framework.

That's all a diagnosis is—a framework. It's reductive by design. It's helpful for treatment. It's helpful to articulate your specific flavor of mental health hardship. It's not helpful for much else. Your diagnosis is not your identity, and making it part of someone's identity is both inaccurate and potentially harmful. I believe the wrong mindset can determine the difference between successful and unsuccessful therapeutic outcomes.

When people become overinvested in their diagnosis, they run the risk of being performative. In other words, even though someone may genuinely have anxiety, if they embrace being anxious as part of their identity, they may conduct themselves in ways that prevent their anxiety from being resolved. For example, maybe someone makes lots of self-deprecating jokes about their anxiety. Perhaps that's their way of explaining what is going on with their mental health without making the topic overly serious. For others, making jokes may become a way to identify as an anxious person. This difference is subtle but important.

It's normal for people to want to be able to explain *why* their loved one is struggling or having difficulties. People often want to see the best in the people they care about, so it's often a relief to be able to point to a diagnosis as an explanation for confusing or undesirable behavior. If someone makes the diagnosis part of their identity, however, they inadvertently make it harder for the people in their life to extend grace and understanding. The diagnosis becomes less of an explanation and more of an excuse. The associated symptoms become a norm, not something someone needs to work on, be responsible for, and have integrity about managing.

I am thinking of a patient named Jacob who told me about a family member, Krista. Krista was diagnosed with something on the bipolar spectrum, much like Taylor Tomlinson. Krista took meds for a while and built a good rapport with a therapist. One of her issues, as far as Jacob—my patient—could tell, was that she used to manage her bipolar disorder by using recreational drugs and drinking lots of alcohol. It was not that she had a serious substance use disorder; she simply didn't want to leave that part of her life behind. Her friends and community liked to stay up all night and party. One of the best things someone with bipolar disorder can do—depending on their symptoms—is to maintain fairly regular sleep patterns. Bipolar disorder can cause people to have excess energy on very little sleep—getting very little sleep can trigger those energetic episodes known as hypomania or mania.

For Jacob, the most difficult part about relating to Krista was not her inconsistent medication usage. My patient's biggest difficulty with Krista had actually nothing to do with her mental illness at all. My patient's biggest problem with her was that everyone allowed her to use her mental illness as an excuse to cause all sorts of problems for others. Krista would gossip or make impulsive decisions that harmed other people. She would cause drama, spread rumors, and take advantage of people. For Jacob, the only thing worse than her behavior was not that she cited her bipolar disorder as a sufficient reason for her actions; it was that nobody held her accountable for her actions. They would hear about her behavior and say things like "You know, she *is* bipolar" and "Krista has *legit* mental issues, though, so it's not her fault."

Krista's behavior can be partly explained by her bipolar disorder, but there is a difference between having a mental illness and taking no responsibility for a mental health concern. Lots of people struggle with bipolar disorder. Lots of people with bipolar disorder struggle to consistently stay on medication. In their defense, medication doesn't always work as well for some as it does for others. This chapter isn't about medication compliance. None of that excuses using your mental health diagnosis to avoid taking responsibility for behaviors. We can have compassion for Krista while acknowledging that she is responsible for her actions and her lack of action when it comes to taking care of herself. In many ways, that is what a mental health diagnosis is for: information on how to take better care of yourself. Whether or not you use that information to your advantage is up to you.

Let me be very clear about something. I have a lot of compassion for people who are on their mental health journey, regardless of where they are on that journey. I don't expect perfection from patients, peers, or even myself. But plenty of people have lifelong mental health diagnoses and accompanying mental health struggles and yet do not use their diagnosis as a way to evade responsibility, morals, or ethics. There is no diagnosis in the DSM for *schmuck*, *putz*, or *jerk*. Even more harmful than people who use their mental illness as an excuse to mistreat others, moreover, are those who enable that same behavior under the guise of mental health awareness and decreasing stigma. It's unhelpful to the person who is being enabled and detrimental to the mental health culture at large.

The dangers of a mental health diagnosis becoming part of someone's identity go further than impeding progress in treatment or being used as an excuse to justify unrelated behavior. Diagnosis is like a framework—like a lens—to understand someone's mental health struggles. When people make it a central part of their identity, they prevent others from seeing them fully. There is so much more to a human being besides their diagnosis. I did not treat Krista, as she was a patient's family member. I only heard about the trouble she caused from my patient's point of view. But I have treated plenty of people with bipolar features, and I can tell you that their diagnosis was the least interesting thing about them. They could be creative, funny, shy, well traveled. One patient I worked with was a polyglot who spoke twelve languages!

As a therapist, it is not simply my job to diagnose, treat symptoms, and then move on to the next patient. Sometimes counseling goals have less to do with diagnosis and more to do with thinking through life's problems or making a big decision. To help patients meet their counseling goals, I have to get to know each individual. I cannot just see their diagnosis. I have to see their personality, their values, their interests, how their interests shape their mind, and all their little quirks and nuances that define categories. I have to do my best to look at them as a person. My worry is that, as mental health gets destigmatized and as more people look at their diagnosis as part of their identity, they will rob themselves and others of that glorious experience of discovering the full extent of their personhood. Just as mental health treatment can take time, learning who you are, discovering who you are becoming, and consciously influencing who you are becoming can also take time. Don't rush that process by clinging to a label that most therapists don't put a lot of stock in, anyway.

> **3 THINGS TO REMEMBER ABOUT MYTH #9:**
> **"YOUR DIAGNOSIS IS YOUR IDENTITY"**
>
> 1. A diagnosis is information about how to take better care of yourself—nothing more.
>
> 2. Your diagnosis doesn't give you a free pass to be a jerk.
>
> 3. There is so much more to a person than their diagnosis.

Myth #10: "You Can Diagnose Yourself"

Lukas made it clear that he was a therapist when he reached out to me for therapy. He knew what he was dealing with but felt stuck. He could not fix his problem himself. Lukas was up-front about his intentions. He only wanted to work with me for a few sessions to figure out his problem so he could take care of his compulsion on his own. At our first session, Lukas disclosed that he had something called trichotillomania, a mental disorder that involved him pulling out his hair. He also picked at his skin—this is called excoriation disorder. He would pick and pick, and many times he would bleed from the excessive picking.

Both trichotillomania and excoriation disorder are grouped together under obsessive-compulsive disorders, sometimes abbreviated as OCD-related disorders. The way you treat typical OCD is by helping the patient identify repetitive and intrusive thoughts: the *obsessions*. Behaviors such as handwashing, skin picking, and hairpulling are understood as compulsive behaviors. Compulsivity, in the context of OCD-related disorders, is understood as actions that help keep the obsessions at bay. For example, if someone has obsessive thoughts about being dirty, they may compulsively wash their hands.

Lukas's frustration was that he picked at his skin and hair at seemingly random times. He felt ashamed to be reaching out to me for help, because he had been to therapy before and liked to think of himself as a self-aware person. He knew the evidence-based protocols for treating OCD. He told me that if he could just have a few sessions with me, he would happily give himself the exposure-therapy treatments. He was paying off his graduate school debt and felt that paying for therapy for a disorder he already knew how to treat was an impractical use of funds.

Here's the thing: Lukas didn't have OCD. I was able to assess through a behavioral analysis that the skin picking and hairpulling were precipitated not by obsessive thoughts but by emotional suppression. It was helpful to understand his behavior as more related to self-harming as a way to deal with unpleasant emotion(s). Some people cut their skin, and others hit themselves, but it's not unheard-of for skin picking and hairpulling to be used as a way to deal with unpleasant emotions or intense anxiety. Lukas was a licensed therapist who diagnosed himself with trichotillomania and excoriation disorder, but he got the diagnosis wrong.

One of the reasons diagnoses matter is that they inform treatment plans. The reason anxiety and OCD are different diagnoses is that they are different things. OCD has obsessions and compulsions, so the treatment focuses on those components. Something like generalized anxiety disorder can have a very different type of treatment. In Lukas's case, he was unaware that following a particularly difficult breakup, he was shutting off his emotions. It didn't happen right away. It started with him picking at his cuticles. As the months went by, the more he suppressed his feelings, the more he picked to deal with the stress. Anxiety is often, but not always, correlated with emotional suppression.

I share part of Lukas's story because I want to be clear that even trained clinicians often have difficulty properly diagnosing themselves. I have sought my own mental health treatment and have found it incredibly helpful. Having said that, I still think it's incredibly difficult to objectively assess and diagnose yourself. In fact, diagnosis is so complex that some psychologists and clinicians specialize in testing and assessment. All they do is see patients, write a report that may or may not include a diagnosis, and then give the report to the patient and the patient's therapist. When I have had patients receive a formal assessment like this, even if they didn't have a diagnosis, I have always found the assessment to be super helpful in formulating their treatment plan.

Personally, I am an *interventionist*. I am a psychotherapist who facilitates psychotherapy, so I do not conduct assessments for a living. I have been trained in the basics of psychological assessment, however, and there are a few things you need to know about this process if you are toying with the idea of diagnosing yourself. First, to properly do an assessment, you cannot just rely on self-reported data. The research is clear: You are not the most reliable narrator of your own experience. The average person's memory is highly subjective, too. In fact, a core part of being trained as a therapist is learning to avoid instilling false memories while being aware that the psychotherapy process will change the interpretation, meaning, and significance of certain memories. People can be highly suggestible, and an important aspect of properly assessing someone is to avoid triggering that suggestibility if possible.

To properly diagnose someone, you have to combine their subjective reports with objective data. This can look like psychological testing, when the clinician might have you fill out certain questionnaires or play certain games while they observe you for data points of which you are unaware. The clinician will also likely call your spouse, your other family members, or your teachers if you're in school. While these interviews are technically subjective, they are helpful because they are about the patient in question but don't come from the patient in question. When it comes to developmental disorders such as ADHD or an autism spectrum disorder, certain features of the diagnosis specify that they have to be exhibited at a young age. It's normal for most people to not remember their childhoods clearly, so interviewing parents is typically quite helpful.

Diagnoses are often critical for informing a treatment plan. If your treatment isn't working, that means one of three things. One, it's too early in treatment to see the benefit, so you need to be patient and press forward. Two, the treatment protocol is ineffective. Three, the diagnosis is *wrong*. Clinicians make mistakes, and anyone has the potential to misdiagnose, but the odds are better if you are not the only one involved in that process. When I suspect that I have misdiagnosed a patient, I am often honest with them about it. I explain that they have more data about themselves than I do, and together we are often able to go back to the drawing board and eventually find something that works. My style of therapy tends to be highly collaborative. Therefore, because the purpose of a diagnosis is to inform a treatment plan, I usually opt to include my patient in that process whenever it's clinically appropriate.

It's also worth noting that it is *possible* to diagnose yourself, but it's not recommended. This is especially true when it comes to diagnosing yourself by relying on social media. One study found that in videos about ADHD on social media, more than half the content is inaccurate or misleading.[1] Another study found that when it comes to autism, only 27 percent of the videos are helpful.[2] In other words, 73 percent of the videos are inaccurate or unhelpful in how they discuss autism. What I recommend to my patients is to use social media to supplement their knowledge but not to replace reading books and research papers or speaking with a qualified professional. There is often no good replacement for therapy. And yet, it is common to see people saying that "self-diagnosis is legit" on social media and being celebrated for it.

Because diagnosis helps inform a treatment plan, therapy can definitely help you with the treatment part of your journey. In Lukas's case, even after I reconceptualized his diagnosis, he stayed in therapy. It is one thing to intellectually understand something, such as a diagnosis. It's another thing to experience the benefits of treatment. The latter cannot always be accomplished by yourself, even if you might be able to diagnose yourself correctly. If you diagnose yourself with something and feel symptom relief promptly afterward, you may not have made the correct diagnosis. Most diagnoses necessitate that the symptoms persist over a certain period of time. Feeling in the dumps for a week and pulling yourself out of it is not the same thing as overcoming major depressive disorder. If you didn't need treatment or help to turn things around, then diagnostic language likely was not actually helpful.

The proliferation and accessibility of all kinds of mental health information have created the unprecedented phenomenon of self-diagnosis. It's an inevitable aspect of the destigmatization of mental health that as the stigma decreases, more people will be curious about whether these labels fit what they are going through. It's understandable: Nobody likes taking the time to go to a doctor's appointment, concerned that something is wrong with their spine, and spending all that time and money, only to be told that they just need to foam-roll their back and stretch more. Therapy can be expensive, so I understand the temptation to consult Dr. Google rather than reach out to someone more legitimate.

I have also noticed that some people who diagnose themselves do not seek treatment, while maintaining that their self-diagnosis is correct. Even though some might be doing this out of economic necessity, many people can afford to go to therapy but choose not to. When I encounter people like this in my life, I get curious about the stages of change. In the precontemplation stage of change, people do not seriously consider changing anything and are not interested in any kind of help or support, professional or otherwise. If that's you or someone you know, the risk of reveling in self-diagnosis is that you are potentially holding yourself back from making changes that could benefit you. Perhaps you know someone who is always using their ADHD as an excuse for missing deadlines, running late, and dropping the ball on priorities. If the person is properly diagnosed, it's reasonable to wonder how well their treatment is working. Does their medication need to be adjusted? Do they need to refresh their executive functioning skills? Or are the symptoms coming from something else and not an underlying neurological difference? If they are self-diagnosed, why aren't they getting the help they need?

Of course, reaching out to professionals can be scary. I always feel a little nervous waiting for test results from my doctor. Maybe you have had unpleasant—or even traumatic—experiences with a previous therapist. Those reservations are legitimate. If you do decide to diagnose yourself, or if you are avoiding treatment for any reason, I hope you carefully consider the points brought up in this chapter. You can lead a horse to water, but you can't make him drink. Even if you pull off the challenging task or correctly diagnose yourself, you can't necessarily change yourself without a little support. That's not just a fact of therapy—that's a fact of life. We're fundamentally social creatures, and we are not good at handling complex issues on our own.

> **3 THINGS TO REMEMBER ABOUT MYTH #10: "YOU CAN DIAGNOSE YOURSELF"**
>
> 1. You cannot diagnose yourself, because people are unreliable narrators of their own experiences.
>
> 2. The craft of diagnosis requires subjective and objective data.
>
> 3. Self-diagnosis may encourage treatment-avoidant behavior.

Part III

Clinical Cacophony: Common Myths About Popularly Misused Therapy Terms

Myth #11: "Everyone Gets Depressed and Anxious"

When people say that everyone gets depressed and anxious, they are usually coming from a good place, but I am not sure that what they're saying is technically correct. If it is correct, I am not sure that it's good for individuals or for society to talk about life this way. When people say that everyone experiences depression and anxiety, the intention seems to be to comfort those who are experiencing difficult feelings. People likely wish to normalize the idea that everyone goes through hard times. While hard times do happen to everyone, these experiences do not need to be labeled as depression or anxiety to be worthy of validation. Hard times can be psychologically impactful without reaching the level of psychopathology. It's much better to encourage supporting people through hard times while working to destigmatize mental illness.

Are people using the term *depressed* when they mean *sad* and the term *anxious* when they mean *worried*? Or have the definitions of anxiety and depression changed over time? This difference matters, because if it's the former, then all we need to do is clarify the definition of these words. If it's the latter, then what does that mean for mental health discourse and mental health culture? If definitions of our mental health–related terms change over time, will that mean more or less confusion when it comes to navigating all this psychobabble?

Concept creep is a term coined by Dr. Nicholas Haslam at the University of Melbourne.[1] It refers to the gradual expansion of definitions of harm-based terms over time to include a wider range of behaviors and experiences. Dr. Haslam is a true researcher; he is careful to avoid either encouraging or discouraging people using his work from making social criticisms or political statements. He does not find concept creep to be good or bad; he simply observes it as a phenomenon to be studied.

Dr. Haslam coined the term *concept creep* in 2016 and has also been studying different words because, naturally, different words may evolve over time in different ways. In 2023, Haslam and his team published a paper called "Have the Concepts of 'Anxiety' and Depression' Been Normalized or Pathologized? A Corpus Study of Historical Semantic Change."[2] In layman's terms, the paper is about exploring whether the terms *anxiety* and *depression* are undergoing concept creep or whether people are just using them interchangeably to describe other normative emotional experiences.

To research this question as objectively as possible, Haslam and his team looked at more than 133 million words from psychology research abstracts published between 1970 and 2018. They also looked at more than 500 million words from various text sources outside the domain of psychology research. Haslam and his fellow researchers hypothesized that the usage of *anxiety* and *depression* would "decline in the average emotional severity over the study period." In other words, Haslam and his team were fans of the normalization hypothesis. They thought that *anxiety* and *depression* were *not* experiencing concept creep. They predicted that people were simply using these words interchangeably with *feeling worried* or *feeling apathetic*.

What the researchers found, though, was the opposite. They write, "The average severity of collocates for both words increased in both corpora." Translating this from researcher speak: The study did not support the hypothesis that over time, the words were being used to describe a broader range of experiences. Instead, the concepts of depression and anxiety themselves have been modified over time so more people and more experiences fit the criteria for depression and anxiety. In other words, what we meant by *depression* or *anxiety* many years ago is different from what we mean by those words today. The definition of the concept expanded, in an example of concept creep.

There are several reasons this could be happening. One could argue that, due to a variety of factors, more people actually are anxious and depressed, which would support the idea that "everyone experiences depression and anxiety" is a fact, not a myth. Different people offer different rationales for an increase in depression and anxiety. Environmentalists argue that the toxins we are exposed to in the air we breathe and the food we eat trigger mental and behavioral ailments. Some social theorists lament the inhumane nature of capitalism, describing depression and anxiety as normal responses to our unnatural conditions. Conservative theorists believe that the slow and steady decay of family values has left the typical human being lost, nihilistic, and mentally afflicted. Others believe that technology meant to connect us—including television, the internet, and social media—has paradoxically left us disconnected from ourselves and from one another, fueling symptoms of anxiety and depression.

Many of these arguments have kernels of truth to them, but I have a few different theories. A broader historical trend is that the average person is more focused on their own emotional well-being than the average person was in the past. The historian James Patterson writes about the cultural revolution of the 1960s in his book *Grand Expectations*. In the 1960s, some Americans began to crystallize their ideas of "rights," while others referred to the same things as "privileges" or "entitlements." Patterson notes, "In personal life, this meant rapid gratification. . . . Some thought that they combat not only the age-old scourges of human life—Disease and Disability—but also two others: Discontent and Dissatisfaction."[3] In other words, in our cultural paradigm, we don't just want to survive—we want to thrive. It doesn't seem to be a coincidence that in 1962, Abraham Maslow presented his ideas of self-actualization and the hierarchy of human needs in his publication *Toward a Psychology of Being*. Maslow hypothesized that when our physical needs are met, we are able to focus on other needs, including belonging, purpose, self-actualization, and more.[4] This is not to say that life in the twenty-first century is perfect and without problems. We still have many problems, including problems with physical needs. But perhaps our fixation on everyone having anxiety and depression is actually a good thing. Because more people are surviving, more people want to thrive.

Another theory is the mental health field tends to pathologize normal behavior. I am not the first to voice this concern. Dr. Allen Frances is a psychiatrist who edited large portions of the DSM-V. In his book *Saving Normal,* he calls out the entire mental health field for failing to maintain boundaries between psychopathology and the normal problems of living that everyone experiences.[5] For example, everyone feels sad and unmotivated when they have a tough time accomplishing their goals. Are they in a low mood because they are clinically depressed? Or is their mood a normal reaction to tough circumstances?

It's not merely a matter of debating semantics or waxing philosophical. It's important that you understand this point, because your own mental health is at risk. For one thing, some research has found that when you apply therapeutic techniques to low or normative levels of anxiety and depression, it can make symptoms worse.[6] For me, this is the biggest reason why we—as a mental health culture—should push back on this idea that everyone gets depressed and anxious. Think about it: If you are depressed because you have suppressed your feelings, then going to therapy and learning to feel your feelings may alleviate your depression. On the other hand, if you are in a slump, think it's depression, and go to therapy, you may wind up ruminating on your feelings instead of processing them in a therapeutic way. If you don't have depression, then therapy might make things worse.

It's tricky to discuss this topic, because I do not want anyone's takeaway to be that their anxiety or depression is not real or worthy of clinical attention. Many people do experience depression and anxiety. I do not want anyone to fear seeking and going to therapy. Any therapist worth their salt should understand how and why their interventions might make things worse. If you are in therapy or curious to try it, you should talk to the clinician about it. Getting on the same page about how to define progress in therapy is always a good idea, and defining how to not make things worse is part of that larger conversation. It's also worth noting that just because you start to feel worse in therapy, that does *not* mean therapy isn't working. Sometimes things feel worse before they get better.

I have worked with many competent clinicians who understand these nuances well. They understand that they do not need to diagnose you with something in order to help you. One of the most effective interventions I have found as a psychotherapist is to *normalize* and not pathologize the patient's experience. When assessed accurately, most people experience huge amounts of symptom relief when they learn that their feelings are understandable, that lots of people worry about these things, and that lots of people struggle in similar ways. It is sometimes less helpful to label their concerns with a scary term such as *social anxiety disorder* when plenty of people feel self-conscious around others or feel nervous speaking in front of a crowd of their peers. Many people enter therapy and are turned off by an overly diagnostic approach. I find that people who are relieved to get a diagnosis really needed the diagnosis, because it named their problem. If you can name a problem, you can fix it. But if the problems you are aiming to fix are problems that everyone experiences, then do you really need therapeutic language to fix them?

I want to end with the following thought: Some therapeutic terms are quite harmful when broadened or misused. I am not sure that *depression* and *anxiety* are at the top of my list of such terms. If someone says they are anxious and what they mean is they are nervous, most people will get that. If someone says that they feel depressed but what they mean is they feel sad, most people will understand them. My issue is that I think the concept creep of these terms makes communication more difficult. I believe we already have the language to describe feeling nervous and feeling sad. If we already have the words to describe what is happening, we should use those words. That way, when someone is dealing with anxiety or depression, we will treat that problem with the seriousness it deserves.

> **3 THINGS TO REMEMBER ABOUT MYTH #11: "EVERYONE GETS DEPRESSED AND ANXIOUS"**
>
> 1. There are many words to describe your internal experience besides *depression* and *anxiety*.
>
> 2. Therapeutic interventions that can help severe depression or anxiety can make normative anxiety and depression worse.
>
> 3. Life has never been and will never be free of sadness, worry, and other unpleasant emotional experiences.

Myth #12: "The Reason You Can't Focus Is ADHD"

I am not sure why social media has so many people thinking they have ADHD. It seems like just yesterday, everyone was concerned that we were overdiagnosing children with ADHD. Today, many people believe they have ADHD, even if they haven't seen a qualified professional. I have spoken to some individuals who claim to have been diagnosed with ADHD and who have been given an accompanying Adderall prescription, but the diagnostic session was only fifteen minutes long. It's not possible to diagnose someone with a neurodevelopmental disorder in fifteen minutes. The problem is that misdiagnosis is not just inaccurate, it's potentially harmful.

What is ADHD? Attention deficit hyperactivity disorder is a neurodevelopmental disorder, which means it's a diagnosis that reflects a difference in how your brain and nervous system developed. The classic symptoms of ADHD include acting without thinking, constantly fidgeting, being unable to concentrate on tasks, excessive physical movement, excessive talking, being unable to wait one's turn, interrupting conversations, and being unable to sit still, especially in calm or quiet surroundings. There are so many nuances to discuss here, but I want to focus on two. First, it's a diagnosis that reflects a neurodevelopmental difference. Second, difficulties with focus and attention are just one aspect of having ADHD. In other words, just because you have disordered attention or focus, that doesn't mean you have a neurodevelopmental difference.

I am fond of this lovely saying about ADHD. I believe it might have been Jason Silva who said it: "These days, if you do not have ADHD, it's because you're not paying attention." I love it because it communicates so much about mental health in a single pithy line with humor and sophistication. Many factors besides your nervous system's development could contribute to having difficulties with focus and attention. In an age of information overload, there are so many things to pay attention to that it can be hard to know what is important and worth giving your attention to. We live in an increasingly complex world; in many ways, Jason Silva's saying normalizes the experience of feeling that we cannot be effective or efficient with our focus.

The first way you know that people are unnecessarily pathologizing their attention, or lack thereof, is that concerns about focus are not a new phenomenon. While we all compete in the attention economy, struggling with focus is a timeless worry. Ancient philosophers discussed the mind's tendency to wander. Medieval monks documented the challenges of *acedia* or spiritual sloth. They struggled with maintaining focus during long periods of study and prayer. Do you really think Leo Tolstoy sat down and wrote *War and Peace* in one fell swoop? It's a safe bet to assume he really wrestled with how to remain focused on such a long manuscript. There's this rumor going around that in the age of social media, everyone has the attention span of a goldfish. So how are we able to binge-watch our favorite TV shows? Why is it that when Joe Rogan releases podcast episodes that are several hours long, he gains the attention of millions of listeners per episode? Although each era of history may have unique factors at play, difficulties with focus are normal and universal, not unique to our current paradigm.

When it comes to issues of focus that *are* a mental health concern, the biggest harm of prematurely assigning the ADHD label is that ADHD does not have a cure. It is one of the few mental health diagnoses for which medication is the first line of defense. That does not mean that therapy cannot help people with ADHD. On the contrary, every single person with ADHD can greatly benefit from learning executive functioning skills from a competent provider. But the right medication and the best ADHD therapist in the world won't be able to help you if you are struggling with focusing for other reasons. If an ADHD diagnosis is inaccurate, you may not be able to get the help you need. If something more serious is underpinning your symptoms, then they may not improve or could get worse.

There are so many other diagnoses that mimic ADHD symptoms. Did you know that some people who are depressed fidget a lot and speak quickly? It's called psychomotor agitation, and it's a feature of depression. Alcohol is proven to impact cognitive performance. It's difficult to stay focused when you're hungover. I don't know about you, but I had a bit to drink on my twenty-first birthday, and I was not the most focused person the next day. You do not need to have a serious addiction issue for substances to be holding you back from optimally functioning. Cannabis or caffeine can cause people to have symptoms mimicking those of ADHD when they "come down" from the high.

Psychobabble

Have you ever tried to focus on something when you're low on sleep? According to Gallup, about one-third of Americans get unsatisfactory sleep.[1] More than half of Americans surveyed use a sleep aid to fall asleep, which could be anything from a white noise machine to medication. Clearly, sleep is a big issue. If you're not well rested or have a sleep disorder, you may have symptoms that completely mimic ADHD. If you had an undiagnosed sleep disorder, would you appreciate it if your mental health care provider prescribed you a stimulant and sent you on your merry way? Or would you benefit from a sleep hygiene protocol that would help you feel refreshed and properly rested instead?

For some people, the dangers can be even more pronounced. When Mikey came to see me, he was embarrassed. He had recently developed certain impulsivity and compulsivity problems. He noticed that a pattern had emerged in which he would make decisions without thinking and had difficulty controlling certain urges to shop, binge on delicious food, and seek out sexual activity. These issues were impacting his professional and personal relationships. For example, he regularly needed to return expensive items from luxury brands that he would purchase online; sometimes the clothes were the wrong size. He was blurting out inappropriate jokes at work and with friends and was noticing people starting to distance themselves from him. Although he had always identified as a sexual person and was comfortable in his sexuality, he noticed that recently he had difficulty controlling his urges. He didn't just want to have sex; he needed sexual release and could not find the patience to wait as he had been able to do in the past. Thankfully, Mikey worked from home, so he could take care of business when his schedule allowed.

I eventually learned that Mikey had started taking Adderall around the time he first noticed the symptoms. He got diagnosed through a company that allowed him to make a convenient telehealth appointment. Adderall treats ADHD, but it's also a methamphetamine. If Mikey had come to you and said some version of the following, what would your reaction be?

> *Hello, mental health professional. I started taking prescribed methamphetamine, which is basically like taking cocaine that lasts several hours. I am coming to see you because I am concerned by my racing thoughts, acting without thinking, and taking lots of risks, and I feel out of control with my sexual desires. What do you think is wrong with me?*

In therapy, sometimes the answers are obvious. My suspicion with Mikey was that he was not benefiting from the Adderall or, if he did have ADHD, was taking way too much Adderall. Taking too much stimulant medication could explain all his symptoms. Mikey did not see the situation that way. I asked whether he was willing to talk to a different prescriber to get a second opinion. I was also concerned that Mikey could have something on the bipolar spectrum. Using stimulants can trigger hypomania, which could also explain many of Mikey's symptoms.

In the end, Mikey was mostly interested in skills and tools I could give him to help him stop being so impulsive and compulsive and keep doing exactly what he had been doing. He didn't want to explore the deeper aspects of his behavior, and he was certainly not in a place to consider giving up Adderall. According to Mikey, while he intellectually understood that stimulant use could cause all the symptoms he was concerned about, the benefits from taking Adderall outweighed concerns about his behavior. I worked with him for a while, but none of the executive functioning tools used to treat ADHD were working. I even tried some behavioral techniques used to treat hypomania, but treating bipolar disorder usually necessitates medication, because it's about stabilizing mood, not primarily about regulating impulsivity.

Eventually, Mikey stopped therapy with me because he wasn't getting the results he desired. I remain curious whether he ever tried stopping the stimulant medication, but I will likely never know. Some people are unwilling to give up the things that are hurting them. When the harm is more subtle or even feels pleasurable—as in Mikey's case—that often makes it more difficult for people to identify the harm, because the consequences are not so obvious. When I reflect on his case, I sometimes wonder whether the enhanced focus, energy, and mood Mikey experienced from the Adderall were worth the downsides. I have trouble accepting that idea, though, because he was in therapy to work on the downsides and was unable or unwilling to rule out his medication as the cause.

---

3 THINGS TO REMEMBER ABOUT MYTH #12: "THE REASON YOU CAN'T FOCUS IS ADHD"

1. Struggling with focus and discipline is a universal and timeless human experience.

2. You may have difficulties with focus for many clinical reasons besides ADHD.

3. If you do have ADHD, medication and therapy can help.

Myth #13: "Mindfulness Is Good for Everyone"

I will never forget one of my first patients, Nancy. I was an intern, so I had been practicing therapy for less than a year. I had assessed that she would benefit from learning to be more mindful, so I guided her through a meditation exercise. As I helped her get super still in her body, I was elated to see that the exercise was working. She was becoming less fidgety, and her breathing was getting deeper and more regular. To my surprise, the meditation culminated in Nancy having a full-blown panic attack right in front of me in the office. I was so surprised that I was not sure what to do next. Sure, I had helped people navigate panic attacks before, but never right after a meditation. When I spoke to my supervisor about the session, she gave me a lesson I would never forget: Mindfulness is *not* good for everyone.

Mindfulness is the practice of being present to, aware of, and nonjudgmental about your internal and external experiences. It's similar to but different from meditation. Meditation is a way to practice being mindful, while mindfulness is a state of being that you can practice in many different settings. Many people mistakenly presume that because mindfulness is helpful for many mental health concerns, it's advisable for everyone to engage in a mindfulness practice.

In Nancy's case, she had a severely dysregulated nervous system. I ended up diagnosing her with borderline personality disorder at a later date, but at the time, she simply presented as anxious. My initial assessment was that being in her body would get her out of her head and lessen her anxiety. The issue was that Nancy had not yet developed the proper emotional regulation skills to handle being that present in her body. She could not be present, aware, and nonjudgmental about her internal emotional experience, because her emotional baseline was one of panic and self-loathing.

If someone has bipolar disorder, being mindful of and nonjudgmental about their emotions is the exact opposite of what they should be doing if they feel a depressive episode coming on. For many people, it helps to judge and fight against the feeling before it escalates into concerning territory. If someone is experiencing psychosis—hallucinating and dealing with delusional thoughts—the last thing they should do is get super present to their hallucinations and delusions. They should actually combat them. When it comes to anxiety or panic disorder, sometimes one of the best things you can do is to distract yourself.

When Nancy learned skills to tolerate high levels of distressing emotions, she would jump into a cold shower and bite into a lemon to distract herself from her panicking mind. If that sounds odd to you, ask yourself whether you have ever felt refreshed after a bath or jumping into a lake or stream. Have you ever eaten ice cream to cope with heartbreak or stress-eaten an entire box of your favorite indulgence to cope with feelings of worry? I bet those things helped you. Nancy's methods were more extreme because her symptoms were more extreme. A cold shower and biting into an overwhelming piece of fruit, like a lemon, helped her because these things were stimulating her physical senses in a way that matched her emotional distress. If I had suggested that Nancy take a bath and eat some Ben and Jerry's the next time she was having a panic attack, she would have likely sought out a different therapist.

We can all learn something very important from Nancy. The strategies that she employed before learning mindfulness—distress tolerance and emotional regulation skills—are examples of *adaptive avoidance*. Sometimes it doesn't make sense to feel your feelings in their deepest expression. Sometimes the best thing you can do for yourself is to avoid your feelings to ensure you do not act on them and make a bad situation worse.

I want to be very clear that I am a big believer in mindfulness. I personally follow a meditation practice that is essential for my self-care and my own mental health maintenance. Sometimes the best way to regulate emotions is to get super present with them and let them pass. It goes back to that old therapy adage: The way forward is through. That's true, sometimes. Other times, it's not going to be the right move to associate deeply into your feelings. It's perfectly normal and healthy to avoid them as well.

One of the curious things I have noticed about the popularization of mindfulness in culture is a movement to help children and young people practice mindfulness. This comes from a desire to raise emotionally resilient children. I have no problem with that goal; in fact, I support it. But I don't think it's a radical statement to point out that part of properly socializing children is to help them suppress certain thoughts, feelings, urges, and desires. Young children need to learn self-control. Have you ever seen a child who is not at the same developmental stage as their peers in terms of emotional regulation? The kind of child who cannot suppress their feelings? This child doesn't have any friends who want to play with them. The kind of psychological damage that causes is much worse than for the child not to have their feelings validated every step of the way. It's okay to care for yourself and your mental health the way you would care for a child you are in charge of raising. You wouldn't let the child just sit in their bad feelings all the time without any comfort—so why are you treating yourself like that?

Like anything else, mindfulness is a tool. Sometimes, it can be helpful. I know it's helped me and many of my patients. But not every tool is appropriate for every situation. Mindfulness is no different.

> **3 THINGS TO REMEMBER ABOUT MYTH #13: "MINDFULNESS IS GOOD FOR EVERYONE"**
>
> 1. Mindfulness is not appropriate for every mental health concern.
>
> 2. It can be perfectly healthy to sometimes avoid feelings or avoid acting on them.
>
> 3. You would never raise a child to just feel everything out in the open regardless of the consequences, so you shouldn't do that, either.

Myth #14: "Your Awkward Friend Is Neurodivergent"

Do you have a loved one or an acquaintance who is awkward, odd, or a little eccentric? Have you ever described them as kind of autistic, somewhere on the spectrum, or neurodivergent? You probably didn't have bad intentions, and your assessment of that person may have been accurate. But did you know that some people use the words *neurodivergent* and *neurodiverse* to signal a political movement?

Dr. Judy Singer is an Australian sociologist who is credited with coining and popularizing the term *neurodiversity*. In an interview posted on YouTube in 2022, Dr. Singer was asked to define the term for everyone.[1] She jokes, "It's a fancy word for all of humanity, but don't tell anyone." Dr. Singer goes on to say that she never actually defined the term but describes "what it was for." She wanted to name a social movement in the mold of the women's movement and the gay rights movement and for "neurological minorities."

Dr. Singer goes on to say that she feels that certain individuals—those who are neurodiverse—are neither mentally ill nor intellectually disabled, but their brains and nervous systems are wired differently. At the end of her talk, she makes a joke: "Isn't everyone on antidepressants?" The crowd giggles with her. She comes across as very likable.

At the same time, her talking points are riddled with inconsistencies. If the word *neurodiversity* is for all of humanity, then why is the movement about neurological minorities? It's worth noting that Dr. Singer is not a clinician; she's a sociologist. She has never treated a single neurodivergent individual in a professional setting. In fact, she's highly critical of viewing neurodiversity as a clinical issue. In her book *NeuroDiversity: The Birth of an Idea*, she writes about the "social constructionist view" of disability. She writes, quite plainly, that disability is a "political issue" because the experience of disability is actually a sign that something is wrong with our social systems; it's an outcome of insufficient social structures that oppress certain individuals.[2] The people she writes about are not disabled in the medical sense, but they are neurodivergent. They would not be oppressed if our social systems met their needs in a more optimal way.

Dr. Singer dedicates whole sections of her book to capitalism, feminist theory, and social justice. In one chapter, she even makes the argument that psychotherapy *cannot* help autistic people. Nowhere—not once—does she mention ways to help individuals who are neurodivergent, unless you count the systemic change she advocates but never clearly defines. While it's reasonable to make an argument for systemic changes that improve a population's mental health, it's disappointing that Dr. Singer does not offer any tangible ways that this change might occur. She offers little to no direction for clinicians who wish to improve their ability to effectively treat this population. She does not make an effort to root her suggestions in our existing scientific knowledge. Not a single section of the book is dedicated to neuroscience, biology, or ways to help or understand neurodivergent clientele. Instead, Dr. Singer finds room to include a section musing on whether or not technology—including the internet and social media—is turning neurotypical brains into neurodivergent ones. Another section encourages and normalizes diagnosing yourself as being neurodivergent.

In some ways, it's okay that Dr. Singer doesn't address these clinical aspects of working with someone who has autistic features or ADHD. After all, she is not a clinician. Furthermore, that is not her point. Her point is to catalyze a social and political movement. What's complicated is that, on the clinical front, I agree with some of what she says. I don't think that some neurodivergent people should be labeled as mentally ill. Dr. Singer makes great points about making accommodations for people who appear high-functioning (sometimes called low-acuity) but may need extra support in times of distress. And viewing a diagnosis such as autism spectrum disorder through a dimensional lens can be helpful for patient care. But because she makes some great points, her other points are often overlooked. Unfortunately, it's not just her reasonable points that have received a lot of attention.

Dr. Singer's beliefs about self-diagnosis and the inefficacy of psychotherapy are wildly popular on the internet. Whether or not you agree with her, Dr. Singer has been massively influential in how everyone talks about autism. Her ideas have spread and have given birth to an ecosystem—a community—of people with whom her work resonates and who create similar and related ideas that then go viral. Online, people encourage one another to self-diagnose. When I have pushed back on the trend of self-diagnosing, I have received comments saying that self-diagnosing is cool. People tell me that I am gatekeeping and harming neurodivergent individuals by doing so. I also regularly receive comments from people rejecting evidence-based practices because these "do not apply" to neurodivergent patients.

I once consulted with a psychologist who specialized in working with neurodivergent individuals. Her thinking was for me to send my patient to TikTok to learn more about themselves. It's important to note that this individual was not diagnosed with anything, by me or another professional. While many neurodivergent-affirming providers would never send their patients to TikTok for psychoeducation, many do, because they agree with Dr. Singer that therapy is harmful for this population. I suspect many of these people view their actions as justified by the politics of the movement itself. They are certainly not justified by any evidence-based practice or ethical code.

If I had to choose only one diagnosis to exemplify the problems with the tower of psychobabble, neurodivergence would be a top contender. How are we supposed to help people who are neurodivergent if they cannot be properly assessed, diagnosed, and studied? Outside of structured studies, how are therapists supposed to learn a cohesive craft if some people are strict with their definitions of autism while others are loose and vague about what does or does not constitute a neurological difference? What happens to other clinical issues that are wrapped up in the neurodivergent label? What about neuroplasticity? What about the evidence showing that early interventions can "cure" autism?[3]

These are not hypothetical concerns. These questions have real-world implications for real people with real mental health struggles. When my patient Oliver came to see me, he was already professionally diagnosed as having autism spectrum disorder. He did not self-diagnose, but he learned a lot about being neurodivergent from the internet. One of the things he learned about was something called rejection-sensitive dysphoria, also known as RSD. The idea is that people with ADHD and autism are extra sensitive to real or perceived rejection. While nobody likes rejection, the internet would have you think that RSD is a condition unique to people with autism or ADHD.

For Oliver, this was coming up in the context of his relationship. He felt that he could not have difficult conversations with his wife because of his RSD. The internet was telling him that his sensitivity to real or perceived rejection would always make confrontations with his wife impossible. I let him know that RSD might be real, but the literature was still very early. His behavior could also be explained by avoidant attachment and being raised to suppress his feelings in a house that punished vulnerability and rewarded stoicism. I assured him that I could help if the latter was the problem. I reminded him that even if his nervous system was wired differently, our nervous systems are plastic. They can change over time.

Within a matter of months, Oliver was able to handle hearing criticisms from his wife without feeling rejected. We accomplished this outcome in two ways. First, we talked about *how* to talk about difficult issues with his wife. Second, I referred him to a trauma specialist. Over time, it became apparent to me that due to emotional abuse he suffered while growing up, Oliver wasn't experiencing RSD—he was being triggered. A variety of interventions culminated in him and his wife being able to have hard conversations about things that mattered. What a shame it would have been if I was a *neuro-affirming* provider and simply enabled his avoidance. What if I had opted to not try to help him because RSD is "hardwired"? The proof that my conceptualization was correct is that the interventions worked.

The funny thing about everyone who feels so passionately about neurodivergent people is this: Is Dr. Singer saying anything new? Didn't we already know that different people have different nervous systems? Isn't it obvious that some nervous systems may be a more natural fit with our social systems than others are? Isn't that why we have accommodations for people who need a little extra support? Isn't it a much more feasible goal to make accommodations more accessible rather than try to redesign capitalism? Most important, isn't the idea that our minds and brains are fixed and cannot be changed the old paradigm of mental illness? Isn't that going backward and not forward when it comes to building a mental health culture that can benefit everyone?

---

3 THINGS TO REMEMBER ABOUT MYTH #14: "YOUR AWKWARD FRIEND IS NEURODIVERGENT"

1. Neurodivergence is a real clinical phenomenon, but many people talk about it as a political and social movement, even if they do not realize they are doing so.

2. Many therapists are part of this movement.

3. Focusing on the social construction of disability runs the risk of preventing people from getting the help they need to improve themselves and their lives without changing the system.

Myth #15: "That Person Is a Psychopath"

Patrick learned to be tough from a young age. He once told me about a childhood memory. It was his first time riding a bike without training wheels and, as children often do when trying to find their balance, he fell. Patrick immediately stood up and, without even dusting himself off, hopped back on to try again. He remembered feeling that it was important to appear fearless. His mother and father were beaming with pride at his resilience and bravery. Nothing could stop their brave little boy.

In therapy, Patrick told me that his ability to suppress his emotions served him well. In his work, he was able to remain logical, even when the stakes were high. His friendships and social life mostly involved golf, a lifelong passion in which he benefited from keeping a level head. One area where his emotional suppression did not serve him well was in his relationship with his girlfriend, who all but insisted he come to therapy or face a breakup. When I asked for details about his girlfriend's concerns, he described a fight in which she became very emotional. She accused him of being cold, like a psychopath. Patrick wasn't sure what she meant but found it upsetting to hear. When she saw how her words distressed him, she calmed down.

Patrick's case was an interesting one, although his story is like that of many men who find themselves talking to a shrink. His emotional suppression was not causing any other mental health problems, from what I could tell, but was certainly causing problems in his relationship. I suggested couples therapy and assured Patrick that I could help him "speak her language" when it came to emotional expression and communication.

Patrick was not a psychopath for suppressing his feelings. Everyone suppresses some of their feelings some of the time. Based on my assessment of him, Patrick had a stoic demeanor and was raised in an environment where emotional expression was not rewarded. He worked in finance, an environment that prioritized being highly logical. When he came to see me, he had never been in a serious relationship before and was not practiced in the art of emotional intimacy.

When Patrick's girlfriend insinuated that he acted like a psycho, what she likely meant was that his stoic demeanor conveyed a perceived insensitivity to her emotional state. Other people use *psycho* to describe people whose behavior is manipulative, immoral, unpredictable, or some type of "crazy." It's a widely used piece of slang that comes from the term *psychopath*. Psychopathy is a well-established clinical phenomenon that has been popularized by slasher films, such as *Halloween* and *Scream*, and by true crime, such as the cases of Ted Bundy and Jeffrey Dahmer. It's worth noting that *psychopath* is not a diagnosis. Instead, clinicians often use the term *antisocial personality disorder* (ASPD).

People who have ASPD share a variety of traits. Below, I have included something called the Hare Psychopathy Checklist, sometimes called the Psychopathy Checklist–Revised (PCL-R). It was initially developed by a Canadian psychologist named Dr. Robert Hare, who has studied psychopaths extensively. I want you to think of someone, or of yourself, and see if this person fits each description none of the time, some of the time, or most of the time. If you want to pretend to be an armchair psychologist, you can mark each item with a pencil. Mark *0* for none of the time, *1* for some of the time, and *2* for most of the time.

- Item 1: Glibness / superficial charm
- Item 2: Grandiose sense of self-worth
- Item 3: Need for stimulation / proneness to boredom
- Item 4: Pathological lying
- Item 5: Conning/manipulative
- Item 6: Lack of remorse or guilt
- Item 7: Shallow affect (a reduction in emotional reactivity)
- Item 8: Callous / lack of empathy
- Item 9: Parasitic lifestyle
- Item 10: Poor behavioral controls
- Item 11: Promiscuous sexual behavior
- Item 12: Early behavior problems
- Item 13: Lack of realistic, long-term goals
- Item 14: Impulsivity
- Item 15: Irresponsibility
- Item 16: Failure to accept responsibility for own actions
- Item 17: Many short-term marital relationships
- Item 18: Juvenile delinquency
- Item 19: Revocation of conditional release (they were kept in jail longer than their "conditional release")

- Item 20: Criminal versatility (they have committed many types of crimes)

I am sure that as you went down the list, you noticed how many people fit at least one or two of the criteria. You may even know someone who fits several different criteria. You may be wondering, *Is this person in my life a psychopath?* Don't worry. To qualify for this diagnosis, you need to score above 30 points based on the scale I gave you (the maximum is 40 points). Even then, it's not always obvious that someone fits the diagnosis. For example, if someone grew up in poverty and committed crimes to stay safe, get fed, and keep warm, would item 18, juvenile delinquency, tend to show they are a psychopath, or not? And if someone is an important businessman or politician, do they actually have an accurate sense of self-worth based on their importance, or did they aspire to that position in society because they had a grandiose sense of self-worth?

Thankfully, if you're not a clinician, you don't need to understand how to parse these possibilities. I am bringing these issues up to help you see not only how tricky diagnosing can be, even for a trained professional, but also how using these terms can be really inaccurate. Some people would find it completely offensive to call a teenager who grew up in the streets a psycho because they fit a few criteria on the PCL-R. Similarly, I believe it's just as unhelpful to label your partner or friend a psycho simply because they *appear* to not be very emotional, like Patrick.

People can be impulsive, shallow, promiscuous, callous, or live a parasitic lifestyle for lots of reasons, and many of these reasons have nothing to do with a mental health condition. It's arguable that some people choose to do bad things because they think they can get away with it, but that is not indicative of a larger pattern or a mental disorder. Just as there is a difference between doing bad things and being a bad person, there is a difference between being a bad person and being mentally ill. Many people who struggle with mental illness strive to be good people, while many people who do not fit the criteria for a mental disorder do bad things.

I am all for humor and exaggeration. I have laughed when someone calls a friend a psycho for acting without much regard for other people's feelings. It's important to remember that if you befriended someone who was a psychopath and you believed them to genuinely be lacking in empathy, you likely would not be keeping them around. You wouldn't be cracking jokes or using the label as a way to get sympathy. You would be thankful that the person didn't cause more damage. You would try to stay as far away as possible. Other types of people—who share just some of the traits of psychopaths—are likely okay people to be around, depending on the situation.

---

3 THINGS TO REMEMBER ABOUT MYTH #15: "THAT PERSON IS A PSYCHOPATH"

1. Psychopathy is a serious and scary psychology to encounter in real life.

2. Many people have traits similar to those of psychopaths, but that doesn't mean these people are psychopaths.

3. It is the combination of traits that make psychopaths who they are, not the presence of a few traits.

Myth #16: "Boundaries Are Just Preferences"

It seems as though every therapist and every person who has been to therapy knows what a boundary is, until they are asked to define it. Here are three definitions of boundaries from three well-known therapists:

> Brené Brown, who has written six number one *New York Times* bestselling books and hosted two podcasts on Spotify, says a boundary is simply "what's okay and what's not okay."[1]

> Esther Perel, whose talks have been viewed by millions, says in her MasterClass on the topic of boundaries, "A boundary is a container so that you know what stays inside, what belongs here in terms of content, material, feelings, information, secrets, you name it. It's a container. And at its best, a boundary becomes a safe container so that I can comfortably live inside of this."[2]

Dr. Nicole LePera, better known as the most popular therapist on Instagram, where her handle is @the.holistic.psychologist, defines boundaries as "rules in a sense, teaching people where our lines [are], where our limits [are], how we want to be spoken to, talked about, talked to, what we're willing to do or not do.... This is a pretty big bag. Essentially, it's where are our limits? How do we want to see ourselves or experience ourselves in relationships?"[3]

Is it just me, or are these three different definitions? Taking a bird's-eye view, many people would say the therapists are all talking about the same thing. To me, the differences matter. If we don't parse out the similarities and differences, we are just building a tower of psychobabble. When I ask colleagues or try to find a poll on what is the central and most important commonality between the different definitions of boundaries, I notice that everyone has a slightly different definition.

I even asked ChatGPT for a definition, just to see whether artificial intelligence could synthesize it in a better way. Here is what I got: "A boundary is a limit or space between you and another person, a clear place where you begin and the other person ends. The purpose of setting boundaries is to protect and take care of yourself. They help individuals to feel safe, respected, and valued." The software proceeded to identify six aspects of boundaries: physical, emotional, intellectual, time, material, and mental. The chatbot could not clearly differentiate between intellectual, emotional, and mental boundaries, even when I prompted it to do so. So even ChatGPT-4o has trouble coming up with a concise and operational definition of this concept that everyone refers to and agrees is important.

Psychobabble

My definition of the word *boundary* combines all the definitions above in a simple way. In order to understand what a boundary is, you need to understand its opposite. The opposite of having a boundary is something called enmeshment. The term *enmeshment* was coined by the seminal family therapist Salvador Minuchin. Enmeshment occurs when two or more different people have such a high level of emotional and psychological involvement that the different individuals lose their senses of self. This situation is considered unhealthy because when people cannot maintain a stable sense of self, they usually end up acting in ways that are detrimental to themselves and, often, to the pairing or the group. For example, a family in which everyone is a planner often won't get much done. A couple who have virtually everything in common will have the same weaknesses and pain points and be unable to help each other. Often, in abusive family systems, a tyrannical parent will demand everyone's conformity, regardless of the physical or mental health consequences.

By contrast, having boundaries means having a sense of self and enforcing that sense of self when enmeshment threatens to produce an unhealthy or detrimental dynamic. Boundaries allow individuals to engage in relationships without losing their sense of self, preferences, desires, quirks, and marks of individuality. The concept goes deeper than simply having differences or different preferences or standards for how you are treated. Boundaries require active enforcement to guard against enmeshment.

I know I am *not* seeing a boundary when someone talks about their preferences but does nothing to enforce them. For example, my patient Quinn had a lot of problems with her friends taking advantage of her. It took a lot of work to help Quinn develop the skills, tools, and self-esteem she needed to communicate her preferences for her friends not to eat snacks out of her pantry without asking and not to show up to her home without letting her know they were coming. Even when she was able to communicate these requests, her friends still ate her treasured snacks and showed up unannounced to hang out. I do not know whether they were doing so to be disrespectful or to take advantage of Quinn's demure nature. I do know that Quinn had to learn to not just communicate her boundaries, but also enforce them. And for Quinn, that meant backing away from these friendships. As she implemented her enforcement, which took the form of shutting the door on people when they showed up unannounced, some of her friends eventually came to respect her boundaries. Others backed away.

Quinn's experience is like that of many different people I have treated or have known in my personal life. That's why my definition of a boundary is one that includes an action. Therefore, it doesn't matter whether your definition is moral, like Brené Brown's, for whom a boundary is "what's okay and what's not okay," or your definition is more like Esther Perel's metaphor of a "container" or Dr. LePera's multidimensional "pretty big bag." You can even prefer ChatGPT's definition of "a limit or space between you and another person . . . to protect and take care of yourself." In my opinion, if you don't reinforce a boundary with an action, then the boundary is not a boundary. It's just a preference that you are not fulfilling.

3 THINGS TO REMEMBER ABOUT MYTH #16: "BOUNDARIES ARE JUST PREFERENCES"

1. *Boundaries* is a widely used but unclearly defined term that is sometimes better articulated as *preferences.*

2. To remember the definition of a boundary, remember that it's the opposite of enmeshment, which involves losing your sense of self in another person.

3. Boundaries are meaningless if they are not enforced, because regardless of the definition, a lack of boundaries will lead to enmeshment, which is detrimental to your mental health.

Myth #17: "People Gaslight You When They Disagree"

In 2022, Merriam-Webster, America's oldest dictionary publisher, made *gaslighting* the word of the year. According to an article from the BBC, searches for the word spiked almost 2,000 percent that year alone.[1] How does this iconic dictionary publisher define *gaslighting*?

Gaslighting is the "psychological manipulation of a person usually over an extended period of time that causes the victim to question the validity of their own thoughts, perception of reality, or memories and typically leads to confusion, loss of confidence and self-esteem, uncertainty of one's emotional or mental stability, and a dependency on the perpetrator."[2]

This is a solid definition. It captures how gaslighting is related to what clinicians call coercive control, a psychological abuse tactic that can be seen in abusive relationships, families, and cults.

Coercive control is behavior or a pattern of behavior that seeks to threaten, humiliate, and intimidate or otherwise abuse another person. While not all forms of coercive control are gaslighting, all gaslighting is a form of coercive control. Gaslighting is a process that takes place over time; it's not something that can happen in one argument. It's a deeply insidious manipulation that can have a long-lasting, but not necessarily permanent, impact on those who experience it.

Interestingly, Merriam-Webster offers a second definition of *gaslighting*: "the act or practice of grossly misleading someone especially for one's own advantage."[3] These are meaningfully different definitions. Why would the dictionary contain such different definitions?

The celebrated author David Foster Wallace, in *Authority and American Usage*, proposed that those who control the definitions of words have undue influence over culture.[4] While that's an interesting theory and may hold some truth, it does not adequately explain why Merriam-Webster would provide two quite different definitions. If the publisher intended to have some sort of cultural influence over all the psychobabble, wouldn't the dictionary editors just pick one definition and leave it at that?

It's my understanding that the task of a dictionary is to provide definitions for how words are used by people in today's culture. One of these two definitions of *gaslighting* is quite specific, because some people use *gaslighting* to mean something specific. That definition is aligned with how clinicians talk about gaslighting as a form of psychological abuse. The other definition is quite general. It's so broad that it makes the term an empty formula, open to subversion. The second definition makes *gaslighting* into a word that people can use to describe lots of different things that are not necessarily akin to psychological abuse. If America's oldest dictionary is providing two different definitions of the term, my guess would be that people are using *gaslighting* in these two different ways. If that's not proof that our culture is rife with psychobabble and misinformation, then I don't know what is.

Ironically, Merriam-Webster's statement on the popularity of *gaslighting* notes that we live in an age of misinformation, which at least partly explains the interest in the word among the general public. If a dictionary does have influence over culture, my contention is that by including both the general and the specific definitions of gaslighting, our dictionaries are actually making psychobabble and psychological misinformation harder to navigate. With tongue firmly in cheek, I have to wonder whether the dictionary's editors realized it would be to their advantage to have the typical person need to repeatedly look up definitions of words. Does that mean that editors are "grossly misleading us for their own advantage"? That's their definition of *gaslighting*, right?

To be clear, I don't actually think that the dictionary is gaslighting us. I share the example to illustrate how easy it is to twist a vague definition to fit almost any circumstance. The problem with people using *gaslighting* to mean "disagreeing" or "being manipulative" is that disagreements and manipulation are ubiquitous and pervasive in every single person's day-to-day life. If a parent misleads their child or teenager for their own advantage, does that count as gaslighting? I am sure a teenager somewhere has already thrown that term at their parents in an argument. If police are interrogating someone who actually did commit a crime and the detective misleads the perpetrator to get them to confess, is that psychological abuse? If someone had murdered my loved one, I would want the police to use every lawful tactic to solve the crime.

I am reminded of my patient Rachel, who sought out my therapy services specifically because she wanted to talk to a man about her boyfriend. Rachel and her boyfriend, Steve, got serious very quickly. They essentially started living together after a few months of dating. While each of them technically had their own place, it was convenient for them to be together most nights out of the week. As their honeymoon phase dwindled, they started to have some communication problems. Whenever Rachel would bring up a difficult topic, Steve would accuse her of gaslighting him. While I was only hearing one side of the story, it seemed to me that it was when they had a disagreement about what was said or what happened that Steve would resort to using this word. I encouraged her to focus less on the definition of the word and more on broaching difficult topics slowly to keep stress levels low.

I eventually suggested that Rachel and Steve try couples therapy, since the source of their distress was certainly a relational issue. My hope was that a good couples therapist would allow them to learn the tools they needed to communicate effectively. As therapists, we're not supposed to have opinions about our patients' partner choices. Of course, we often do. While it's possible to prevent your opinion from interfering with the therapy, it's difficult to not have an opinion at all. I didn't love how Steve was using therapy-speak, but I also knew that Rachel really cared about him. At one point, the couples therapist wanted to speak to me, so both Steve and Rachel signed a release of information granting permission for us therapists to discuss the couple's case. I was surprised to hear that Steve didn't bring up gaslighting one time in couples therapy. My theory is that Steve was using the term defensively and reactively to avoid talking about difficult topics that were likely emotionally activating for him. I have a lot of sympathy for Steve. Lots of people, myself included, have behaved in ways they are not proud of when they get scared while navigating a new and intimate relationship. I don't think he was manipulating Rachel or being malevolent. I do think he was using a therapy-related term to throw up a wall. While doing so was misguided, it was certainly understandable.

All this psychobabble around the term *gaslighting* is harmful on two counts. People can use this word to avoid leaning into intimacy, as Steve did. The loose definition of the term also harms the survivors of gaslighting. When people use *gaslighting* to mean "disagreement" or "manipulation," they obscure the brutal and disorienting experience that gaslighting is for those who experience it.

When Taylor came to see me, he immediately showed signs that he was currently being gaslit by a significant other. Not everyone who experiences gaslighting develops the same psychological symptoms. Gaslighting is not a diagnosis, and it can actually result in multiple types of traditional diagnoses. While I wasn't initially certain that what Taylor was experiencing was gaslighting, Taylor second-guessed himself in most of what he shared with me, beginning with our first session together. He had super low self-respect and high levels of anxiety, and he constantly apologized when he felt that he'd misspoken.

When someone important to you works hard to get you to

mistrust your own perception of reality, it works. That doesn't make survivors of gaslighting weak or flawed—it makes them human. Think about it this way: If you remember someone saying something at a dinner, but six of the other dinner guests correct you, the normal thing to do is to assume you misremembered what was said. Human beings are deeply social creatures. If the person you are intimate with disagrees with you, the least you can do is consider that their perspective might be accurate. That's a normal reaction. The issue is that someone who is gaslighting you disagrees with you strategically, over time, to bring you to a place psychologically where you can't trust your own thoughts about yourself.

Taylor was in that headspace when he came to see me for therapy. The gaslighting was so severe that his partner would rearrange their living room furniture and insist that the furniture had always been arranged like that: "You really need to see someone about your memory, Taylor. I am getting concerned." The gaslighting hadn't started that way; months of mind games eventually led to Taylor doubting his reality. It started with small things, but before he knew it, Taylor wasn't sure whether or not the furniture really had always been arranged that way.

Treating a survivor of gaslighting is delicate work, especially if they are currently being abused in that way by their partner. You cannot simply tell them that their perception of their partner is incorrect. That would literally be engaging in behavior that feels similar to the gaslighting the survivor is experiencing. Instead, you create a safe space where they can speak their truth, disagree with you without fear of punishment or pushback, and slowly build up their self-respect so they can defend themselves again.

I vividly remember the day Taylor started to become conscious of his situation: "I think I've been getting lied to for a very long time," he said. In many ways, that's when our work really began. Taylor is doing better now. He was able to stop living with that person and had a long single period before he dove back into the world of dating.

I think of Taylor and cases like his when I hear people joke about gaslighting at a party or use the term to refer to a politician or someone they don't like on TV. I don't think most people would use that word if they knew Taylor's story—do you? Some people hear his story and assume he is weak-minded or should have caught on sooner. I would remind those people that when we are sexually and romantically attracted to someone, it is difficult to see them clearly, especially at the start of the relationship. Everyone should be educated on what the grooming process is like for gaslighters, just as everyone should know the warning signs of cult indoctrination. Many people who exit cults try their best to explain that they're not stupid; they just trusted the wrong person. Survivors of gaslighting are no different. Gaslighting can happen to anyone, and misusing the term, expanding the definition to mean all sorts of things, doesn't do a thing to prevent more people from falling for it. In fact, using the term so loosely likely confuses a lot of people and increases the chances that they might overlook the signs of actual gaslighting.

So the next time you think about using the word *gaslighting* in jest or in exaggeration, consider the disservice you may be doing to someone who doesn't know what you know.

> **3 THINGS TO REMEMBER ABOUT MYTH #17:
> "PEOPLE GASLIGHT YOU WHEN THEY DISAGREE"**
>
> 1. *Gaslighting* is a widely used term with both a specific definition and a vague one.
>
> 2. The vague definition is harmful because it obscures the real danger and harm of gaslighting and how it impacts people.
>
> 3. You can disagree, manipulate, or even abuse others without gaslighting them in the technical sense of the term.

Myth #18: "Your Ex Is Definitely a Narcissist"

Are you familiar with the work of Dr. Ramani Durvasula? It is my opinion that few other mental health professionals have had such a profound impact on how we talk about narcissism. She is a licensed clinical psychologist. Her YouTube videos and social media clips are so prolific that she easily reaches millions of people. Her latest book, *It's Not You: Identifying and Healing from Narcissistic People*, was an instant bestseller.[1] While other people have built brands around discussing narcissism, few have been as successful as Dr. Durvasula. As a mental health culture, we owe her credit for making information about narcissism accessible. But she also deserves credit for making many people misunderstand and misuse the term *narcissism*. As a trained mental health professional, I do not believe her talking points always hold up to scrutiny.

What is narcissism? If you ask Dr. Durvasula, she is usually careful to clarify that she is *not* talking about narcissistic personality disorder (NPD). According to the DSM-V, NPD is a chronic condition characterized by a pervasive pattern of grandiosity, need for admiration, and lack of empathy. Narcissists are often highly exploitative, demand excessive admiration, and believe they can only be understood by or associate with high-status people or institutions. Narcissists are entitled, arrogant, haughty, and often believe others are envious of them.

Dr. Durvasula isn't referring to a diagnosis. She is talking about a personality style or pattern. In her inaugural TEDx Talk on the subject, she mentions Dr. Allen Frances, a psychiatrist who helped formulate the classification of NPD for the DSM.[2] In his book *Saving Normal,* Frances urges people to avoid medicalizing bad behavior. If you ask him, not every bad person is mentally ill.[3] I agree with him. So does Dr. Durvasula. In her TEDx Talk, she describes how narcissism is a normative—and dangerous—personality trait. She says it's just like being extroverted, agreeable, or stubborn; it's *not* something a person can change. It's this illusion of redemption that keeps people in abusive relationships with narcissistic people. She says that pushing back on narcissism is a "human rights issue." Essentially, for Dr. Durvasula, dealing with narcissism is an issue of social justice.

She does not contradict the DSM-V definition of narcissism, but she broadens and adds to it. She writes about how narcissists are always fragile and insecure and their narcissistic traits are maladaptive attempts to cope with their underlying shame. She talks about how there are different kinds of narcissists: grandiose narcissists, vulnerable narcissists, communal narcissists, self-righteous narcissists, neglectful narcissists, and malignant narcissists. While they may come in different flavors, they all have the same source: a fragile ego running from itself and getting what it needs by using and abusing others.

Dr. Durvasula is smart, well-spoken, and convincing. Even I have to admit that I have learned a lot from her videos. One of my favorites is called "The Best Way to Deal with Narcissists Without Arguing."[4] I found this video helpful. But as someone who is a trained professional, I have some questions about her main talking points. For example, she simultaneously insists that she is not talking about a personality disorder but then describes the personality *style* as rigid, fixed, occurring across contexts, and always leading to relational dysfunction. That is exactly how the DSM classifies a personality disorder. It seems that she wants to claim that she's not talking about personality disorders but then defines the narcissistic personality as disordered.

Dr. Durvasula is careful to include a section in her book about how, if we overuse or misapply the term *narcissism*, we risk diluting the term's "potency." She clarifies that just because someone is a jerk, unfaithful, or self-centered, that does not make the person a narcissist. At the same time, she also says that she is not concerned with being precise because when people get lost in the debate over what does or does not constitute narcissism, they stay in narcissistically abusive relationships. She says that "being clear on narcissism may actually muddy your own waters." She adds that "moderate narcissism" is the focus of her book *It's Not You*.

So which is it? Are we going to be precise about applying the narcissism label so that we preserve the term's potency? Or are we going to discuss "moderate narcissism" more generally? If we are going to discuss the moderate part of the narcissism spectrum, then I wonder why she is not using her platform to clarify that all of us exist on this spectrum of narcissism. Most of us have sprinkles of narcissism in our personality. In contrast to the

DSM-V definition of narcissistic personality disorder, normative narcissism means that everyone has some need for validation and some level of self-interest. While some people are more narcissistic than others, that does not mean they have a personality disorder. It also does not mean they are rigid in the way she describes. I cannot find a good example of her acknowledging that narcissism is common and may even be acceptable. In fact, she paints a picture in which many of us are not narcissistic ourselves but are abused by narcissists in our relationships. She speaks as a guest on podcasts and says things like "one in six people are narcissistic."[5] She thinks that 40–50 percent of famous people and 60–70 percent of world leaders are narcissistic.

First of all, these statistics she is sharing are just guesses with no basis in fact. More important, these statistics are lacking important context about how narcissism works. Dr. Durvasula fails to clarify that many writers on the subject of narcissism believe that moderate amounts of narcissism in someone's personality can be a *good* thing. People who are ambitious—who feel they are entitled to success and believe they are special and can be good leaders—often become the changemakers and leaders the world needs. Dr. Durvasula actually hints at the helpful aspects of moderate narcissism when she says in an interview with Steven Bartlett, "I wish I was more grandiose because my career would be fire, but I'm not."[6]

Interestingly, she is admitting that grandiose coping styles are not just normal but can actually be beneficial. I would argue that grandiose coping styles are healthy if they are helping you function and achieve your goals in an adaptive way. What is a grandiose coping style? Everyone feels insecure sometimes. When people get insecure, they either one-down or one-up themselves.

For example, maybe someone asks a person on a date and gets rejected. If the person tends to one-down themselves, they might have thoughts like *I will never be good enough* and *It's so much easier for everyone else to date than it is for me*. This is an example of an insecure coping style. On the other hand, other people one-up themselves. They have thoughts like *That person is just intimidated by me* or *It's just really loud in here—if we were somewhere quieter, this person would be more into me*. This is an example of a grandiose coping style.

My problem with Dr. Durvasula is not that I think she is a mouthpiece of misinformation about narcissism. On the contrary, I think more of what she says is true than is untrue. But she offers a perfect example of how psychobabble can lead to more confusion and less understanding—with real-world consequences. I am thinking of my patient Uma. When Uma came to see me, she made it clear that she was ready to do "the work" and to be in therapy. She came to therapy because of the way her last relationship had ended. Her ex-girlfriend had given her the feedback that Uma was very narcissistic and needed to work through that in therapy. Uma was sheepish about this feedback when she told me about it. I remember clearly that she immediately confessed that other exes had given her similar feedback, so naturally, she thought there might be some merit to it. Of course, everyone, including Uma, should take their exes' reviews of them with a grain of salt— that person is your ex for a reason. At the same time, Uma wanted to improve her ability to be in an intimate relationship, and she was hopeful that therapy could help.

Most experts—including Dr. Durvasula—generally agree that narcissists rarely sign up for therapy at all, let alone go to a therapist to work on their narcissism. I sometimes wonder if that's changing with all the public awareness about narcissism. Nevertheless, I started to assess Uma and eventually referred her to a specialist. I had a hunch that what was going on with her wasn't narcissism, and I was right. Uma was somewhere on the autism spectrum. While Uma did not meet the full criteria, the testing psychologists agreed that Uma likely had differences in her nervous system. The "lack of empathy" that Uma's exes observed could have been explored with curiosity, if the exes had been trained professionals. Instead, they jumped to conclusions and ended the relationship instead of understanding that, sometimes, people with autism don't express empathy in an obvious way. They have a different kind of nervous system, in which empathy is facilitated differently.

When you observe someone's narcissistic behavior, I want you to approach it with curiosity, the way I did with Uma. Here's the thing: You may be correct that you are observing narcissistic behavior—but that's not enough. You need to be curious about why the behavior manifests as it does. Exploring this question will allow you to consider other explanations and get at the truth. The truth is important, because if a person is rigidly narcissistic, that's probably something you want to know, isn't it? And if something else is actually going on, you probably want to know about that, too. The truth is that psychology is not very old compared with other fields. There are many compelling and competing perspectives out there.

My favorite challenge to modern discourses on narcissism is found in a book that many therapists have read, but nonclinicians may not have encountered. In her famous book *The Drama of the Gifted Child*, Alice Miller makes the argument that grandiosity and depression are two sides of the same narcissistic coin.[7] Miller tells the story of a young man who was a sensitive and perceptive child. Due to his temperament, he felt immense pressure to meet the emotional needs of his parents. This dynamic led to a loss of the boy's authentic self, as he learned to suppress his own needs and feelings to gain parental approval and love. The boy was able to suppress the torture of having his feelings invalidated and discounted. His personality became a grandiose one. Throughout his life, he continuously achieved. He excelled at sports, dated beautiful women, and always showed off his charm and his brilliance. For a while, this worked. But, tragically, his personality structure had no real foundation. As he got older, the reality of his childhood became unescapable. He experienced bouts of depression but could escape them through swings of grandiosity, fueled by additional achievement. Over time, his achievements—rooted in unhealthy narcissism—were less and less effective at fending off depression, as if he developed a tolerance to a drug.

This man's narcissism was unhealthy because his achievements were not rooted in authenticity. Miller explains that the only way to escape the depressive cycles is to escape grandiosity that staves them off. The man was able to shift into a healthier narcissism only after he mourned the loss of his childhood. Miller explains that his grandiosity shielded him from pain—but the opposite of depression is not an existence without pain. The opposite of depression is an existence in which you have the "freedom to experience spontaneous feelings." When the boy achieved things to suppress his feelings, he had to keep on achieving to avoid the pain. Miller is careful to explain that those who remain depressed and never cycle into grandiosity are not less narcissistic. They still believe they can achieve their parents' love by suppressing their feelings. They also believe they can be inauthentic and win people's affection. These individuals just go about things in a different way from the grandiose types.

Miller's analysis is considerably more compassionate than the views of many on the internet who seek to educate the public about narcissism. Miller's analysis also still applies to interpretations of phenomena such as vulnerable narcissism, in which the individual is narcissistic without being grandiose. Of course, I do not want to imply that all that unhealthy narcissism is acceptable or that we should excuse narcissistic behavior just by understanding its roots. I just think that if we are going to accept someone's depression rooted in suppressing feelings, then we can consider accepting low to moderate levels of narcissism and grandiosity. First of all, I believe that sort of narcissism is curable, if you want to think of it as an illness. Second, I don't think it's a ridiculous claim to say it's ethical to show such individuals compassion, because, as I have said, we are all a little narcissistic. If you are going to speak on the topic, you need to be able to admit that fact, not only about yourself, but about humans in general.

Maybe your ex *was* a narcissist or at least had some narcissistic traits. Or maybe that's just how your ex handled the stress of the breakup. In the wake of a breakup, it's normal to one-up yourself and get a little grandiose. I know I have responded to a breakup that way. It's normal to look at your ex as *the worst*, at least temporarily. That's a normal part of the processing of your separation. Is it easier to view your ex in a balanced way and consider that all their actions and opinions and perspectives are also valid? Is that helpful for you, when what you really need to do is find the motivation to move on? As long as you're not rigid about it, I would argue that adopting the grandiose coping style is way healthier. You can view your ex from a more balanced perspective when you have had time to reflect on the relationship.

I am reminded of the words of Nancy McWilliams: "I have always been more interested in exploring individual differences than in arguing about what is and is not pathology."[8] In the essay those words are from, McWilliams dedicates her energy to being better able to help different kinds of people with different kinds of personalities. For many therapists, that is the goal when they depart from precise and diagnostic criteria: to understand individuals more deeply. My hope is that as you try to develop a deeper understanding of your ex, your parents, or yourself, you approach this work in the spirit of thinkers such as McWilliams and Miller, and not by simply repeating the sound bites you get from the internet.

> **3 THINGS TO REMEMBER ABOUT MYTH #18:**
> **"YOUR EX IS DEFINITELY A NARCISSIST"**
>
> 1. Having a grandiose coping style is not the same thing as being narcissistic.
>
> 2. The more rigidly narcissistic you are, the more likely you are to have NPD.
>
> 3. Narcissism and grandiosity can be "cured" in their mild to moderate manifestations, but that doesn't mean you should stay with someone who is mistreating you.

Myth #19: "I Am a People Pleaser Because I Defer to You"

My grandfather is known for his wise and pithy advice. While he's technically my step-grandfather, I don't think of him that way. He's my "Pops." Pops is from Mexico, and his words of wisdom are often delivered in a straightforward and machismo package. When I was younger, I remember sitting with Pops and Nana as they watched television. I want to say it was *Law and Order*, because that was frequently on television when I was at my grandparents' house. When Nana asked Pops for the remote, he handed it to her and allowed her to change the channel in the middle of the episode. That's when he looked at me and said, "Mijo, see how I just gave her the remote? That's how you love. It makes her happy, and it's not a big deal."

My grandfather is a man of few words, so when he does speak, I make sure to listen. As a therapist, I appreciate the sophistication of his insight. He is basically saying that when you like someone, you want to make them happy. Typically, you make people happy when you defer to their needs, wants, and preferences. This can be about something small, like what to watch on television or what to get for dinner. It can be about something a little more significant, like where you and your partner get married or where you two will spend your one week of vacation time a year. It can even be about serious decisions, like converting to a different faith or staying in a job you resent because you can better provide for your loved ones.

Are people who make decisions to make others happy or provide stability to a relationship people pleasers? I don't think so. My understanding, as a therapist, is that people-pleasing signifies a harmful pattern of behavior that is detrimental both to the individual who is people-pleasing and to the dynamic of the relationship in question. Specifically, if the people-pleasing leads to significant stress, burnout, and resentment, then perhaps the people-pleasing was not coming from a place of love and a desire to positively impact the relationship. Maybe it was coming from a place of fear, where the person is afraid the relationship cannot handle any conflict through disagreement. Sometimes, people-pleasing comes from a place where individuals have such low levels of self-respect, they do not believe they deserve to get what they want, so they don't bother trying to get it.

As one viral meme trend has put it, "Oh, you're a people pleaser? Name one person who is pleased with you." This humorous take signals what I think is wrong with the term. It's not that the phenomenon is not real, but it's a misnomer. I don't think we should call people pleasers by that name, because it misses the point and robs people of the opportunity to own what's actually going on in their relationships. For example, if the person is a doormat, martyr, enabler, or approval seeker, we can call them whichever one of those terms applies. These terms give us more data about what is actually happening. A doormat needs to learn to stand up for themselves. A martyr needs to stop self-sacrificing when no one asked that of them. Enablers avoid conflict to the detriment of others, and approval seekers are inauthentic in terms of what they actually think, believe, and enjoy.

If someone is codependent, then the goal of their therapy should be to become more independent or interdependent. If someone is overaccommodating, they need to develop skills and tools to be less accommodating. If someone is a yes-man or a yes-woman, is this even a problem if it's not leading to any detrimental outcomes? If the person is highly agreeable in terms of their temperament and simply prefers other people to make decisions, then maybe they are not "people pleasers"—maybe we can leave them be. If they are truly self-aware of their temperament and happy with it, I see no issue. Even low levels of conflict cause some people stress. These types of people do well to be selective about whom they displease, because doing so will take more out of these individuals than it would out of someone who is more disagreeable, who is energized by conflict.

As I write this, I am noticing the sheer number of labels we have for this pattern of behavior: people pleaser, doormat, codependent, martyr, enabler. . . . While I wholeheartedly believe that precision in using these labels would be far more helpful, I also wonder whether we should resist allowing people to identify with this behavior. If it is detrimental to them and others, we should encourage people to integrate their deeper motivations in an adaptive way. Instead of saying that the person is an enabler, maybe say that the person is someone who enables others a little too often, and they should keep an eye on that. I know I must sound like such a therapist writing this: It's not that you *are* a people pleaser, it's that you *have* people-pleasing tendencies. I sincerely believe that words shape the meaning of our lives, and it's important to be thoughtful about how we talk about one another and ourselves. A people pleaser is wired that way; a person who engages in people-pleasing behavior has agency and flexibility to change.

Interestingly, I find that many therapists are more agreeable than not. This observation makes sense. If the average shrink thrived on conflict and disagreement, they likely would have picked a more competitive profession instead of one in which you constantly "yes and" your patients every time they resist your interpretation. If the stereotype is true, then it's worth pointing out that many people feel quite emotionally close to their therapist. Many therapists understand that if we want our patients to feel close to us, we are often going to want to defer to them.

Much like my Pops, many therapists and many people find a lot of meaning in giving others what they want. Of course, this is different from saying yes to things you desperately want to say no to because of some underlying psychological pattern. I don't know about you, but I like being and feeling close to the people in my life. Therefore, I am not going to overthink my agreeable tendencies with them. If they want the remote, I will give it to them. There's absolutely nothing wrong with that.

> **3 THINGS TO REMEMBER ABOUT MYTH #19:**
> **"I AM A PEOPLE PLEASER BECAUSE I DEFER TO YOU"**
>
> 1. *People-pleasing* is a broad term that is often misused and misapplied.
>
> 2. When possible, use other terms to more accurately describe the dynamic of a relationship.
>
> 3. Deferring to others is not a sign of a mental health concern, unless there is some sort of notable detriment to an individual and their relationships.

Part IV

Trauma Drama: Common Myths About Trauma

Myth #20: "Everyone Has Trauma"

Trauma is real, but that doesn't mean that everyone has trauma. Many mental health advocates and professionals, in a good-faith attempt to normalize life's difficulties, say that everyone has trauma. This is not true. We need to get on the same page, as a mental health culture, about what trauma means so we can properly study it, treat it, and disseminate proper information about it. If everyone has trauma, then trauma is meaningless as a distinction. Instead of saying that everyone has trauma, it may be much more helpful to say that everyone feels unpleasant emotions and experiences difficulties in life, such as stress, loss, grief, and tragedy.

It is my contention that those who are unwilling to be critical of trauma discourse may be doing more harm than good. People who are unwilling to be critical or thoughtful about how we use and misuse this word, in my opinion, move mental health acceptance backward, not forward. They may be unintentionally doing more harm to survivors of trauma, not less, and are certainly compromising research on trauma and trauma treatment. These people participate in the psychobabble that risks making the project of building a sustainable mental health culture completely untenable.

TRAUMA VERSUS HARDSHIP

It is vital that we normalize the differences between trauma and normative hardship. The word *trauma* comes from a word that means "wound." For example, a trauma surgeon would be the one to treat you if you got into a car accident. If you developed PTSD from this car accident, you might need to see a trauma therapist. Not everyone needs surgery after an accident, and not everyone needs therapy. Just because you experience hardship in life, that doesn't mean you've developed trauma that requires clinical attention. Furthermore, when we say that everyone has trauma, we are inadvertently saying that those who struggle with trauma diagnoses don't deal with anything different from what the rest of us deal with. This is not true. Anyone who has been trained to treat trauma or to interact with sexual assault survivors, domestic abuse survivors, or veterans knows that PTSD is very real. Those who survive the disasters of war, earthquakes, and car accidents know that processing their trauma can be a completely different experience from processing other experiences of stress or tragedy.

TRAUMA VERSUS STRESS

Dr. Robert Sapolsky at Stanford University has a great definition of physical stress. He distinguishes between a stressor and a stress response. A stressor is anything that knocks your body out of homeostasis. Your stress response is your body's attempt to return to a baseline. In his book *Why Zebras Don't Get Ulcers*, Dr. Sapolsky uses as an example of a stressor a zebra's experience of seeing a lion on the savanna.[1] The zebra's physical response to seeing the lion is the stress response: being flooded with adrenaline and running away from the lion to feel safe again. When someone develops something like PTSD, what we mean is that they have developed a trauma response to a certain stressor. The stressor (seeing a lion) leads to a response in that individual (the trauma). In the DSM-V, PTSD is classified as a "trauma and stressor"–related disorder—which makes me wonder whether the conflation of trauma and stress in cultural discourse about trauma is actually the fault of those in the mental health field.

The key difference between trauma and stress is that while all trauma responses are like stress responses, not all stress responses are trauma responses. In other words, we can experience stress without developing a trauma response. I can get stressed by seeing a lion on a hike, but I may not develop PTSD, unless the lion attacks me. Sapolsky talks about how our nervous systems cannot always tell the difference between a real danger and an imagined danger. Biologically, our nervous systems respond to the stresses of the modern world—for example, forgetting to reply to your boss's email—the same way a zebra would respond to seeing a lion. In these situations, you and the zebra would experience increased adrenaline, though you would likely experience less adrenaline than the zebra running for safety would. Once your body remembers you are physically safe and your adrenaline decreases, you would likely feel calm enough to respond coherently to the email.

TRAUMA AND SUBJECTIVITY

When people learn about the subjective nature of stress and trauma, they not only think that everyone has trauma, but they also believe that anything can be traumatic, because trauma responses are subjective. When people learn that trauma responses can be subjective, they are agreeing to the presupposition that events themselves are not traumatic. Instead, our responses to them can be representative of a trauma response. That's how trauma responses are subjective. In other words, trauma is not a way to describe an event, but an individual's response in trying to process that event. The research has shown that different people can experience the same event, and one person will develop PTSD and another will not. Two people can get into the same car accident, or two soldiers can go fight in the same war, yet one of them develops PTSD while the other one is fine.

I don't think people should say "I have trauma" or "I got trauma from that car accident." We should say, "I have a trauma response that I haven't healed from yet." Framing events this way lends to a certain level of implied resiliency and individual agency. Many therapists already engage in such a practice with other diagnostic and subclinical language. People are survivors, not victims. Our patients are not depressed, they *have* a depression-related diagnosis. Our patient is not borderline, they *have* a personality disorder. Furthermore, describing events as inherently traumatic misses the fact that trauma responses vary among individuals. This further confuses discourse about trauma and how trauma responses vary between different people and different populations.

TRAUMA VERSUS PTSD

You might wonder whether trauma symptoms still count if someone does not meet the formal criteria for PTSD. I would say yes. Of course your trauma response is still worthy of clinical concern even if you don't meet the full criteria of PTSD. Although I could not find studies of those who develop trauma-like symptoms to being in war zones and car crashes, I am sure that there are many people who would benefit from trauma therapy without checking every single box of the PTSD checklist. But if you get into a car crash and you find yourself feeling nervous getting into a car again, does this count as a trauma response, or are you engaging in avoidance behavior? If your anxiety doesn't impact your behavior or functioning in any way, does that mean you are experiencing a trauma response? If people are affected and impacted by something that happened to them, they can talk about it as such. They can say they feel "shaken up," "nervous," and "scared" to get into a car again. But if they are not engaging in avoidant behavior—an example of a symptom in many trauma responses—then I don't think they should claim to have a trauma response. Anyone can feel shaken up after a car accident, but not everyone experiences a trauma response. Just because trauma responses are subjective, that doesn't mean any impact from an unpleasant event can be classified as a trauma response. This is—admittedly—a confusing concept.

The consensus of the mental health field used to be that trauma was valid only if it was textbook PTSD. Then we moved on to a more dimensional model of trauma, which assumed that individuals could have some PTSD symptoms but not all of them. Then there was this concept of "big T" versus "little T" trauma. Big T trauma might involve being in a war or being in a plane crash. Little T traumas are trauma responses to little things like falling off your bike or being embarrassed in public. Personally, I am not sure why we differentiate big and little traumas if the trauma response criteria is the same. This is yet another example of why it's important to normalize that there is nothing traumatic about an event in itself; trauma is our response to an event. When this is emphasized, we don't need to clarify whether a trauma response involved big or little trauma—both are clinically valid.

In my opinion, it's a trauma response if your nervous system has organized itself to deal with the traumatic event in question in ways that we know are indicative of trauma. Maybe you avoid reminders of the event. Maybe you're hypervigilant and look for reminders in everything. Maybe you have intrusive memories. Maybe you develop unhelpful, maladaptive beliefs to prevent the traumatic event from happening again. The message here is that just because trauma responses are subjective, that doesn't mean every response is a trauma response. Remember: While all trauma is a stress response, not all stress is a trauma response.

---

3 THINGS TO REMEMBER ABOUT MYTH #20: "EVERYONE HAS TRAUMA"

1. While all trauma is a stress response, not all stress is a trauma response.

2. Trauma is a way to describe your response to an event, not the event itself.

3. Just because trauma responses can be subjective, that does not mean that anything can be classified as a trauma response.

Myth #21: "Trauma Is the Same Thing as Grief"

When I was eleven years old, my father died on a family vacation to Disney World. He died in his sleep, from an undiagnosed heart condition. I was sharing a bed with him at the time. My younger brother was in the other bed with our mom. I was woken up to my mother throwing the blankets off me and telling me to go get help. I remember the policeman who took us to the hospital drove slowly, despite there being nobody on the road so early in the morning. I will never forget the look on the doctor's face when he came into the room to tell us he was gone. He didn't have to say a word. When he walked in, I just knew. I remember feeling frightened and crying a lot.

I developed a series of diagnosable mental health conditions in response to my father's death. I dealt with panic attacks and depression. I developed a trauma response to his passing. In hindsight, I can identify different trauma symptoms even years after his death. One example was how I navigated intimacy with men. Putting romantic interests aside, I engaged in a lot of avoidant behavior in my friendships with men. When I was in college, I swam and played water polo, and I always opted to share a hotel room with the girls during an away tournament. It's incorrect to assume I made that choice because I am gay; there were plenty of gay men on the team. I believe it was trauma. Part of my journey has been letting my walls down around men. Dating men and developing close friendships with people on my sports teams and in my college fraternity were essential to my healing process.

When my dad died, I also dealt with grief. I still deal with it. It's important to distinguish between grief and trauma because they are two fundamentally different concepts. The difference is not just a matter of semantics. It has implications for how we can help ourselves—and our loved ones—move through the inevitable suffering in our lives. Distinguishing between grief and trauma is important so we can learn how to appropriately process both. In trauma, we typically see beliefs develop about ourselves, others, and the world to attempt to prevent the trauma from happening again. Helping these beliefs become more adaptive is key to overcoming the trauma symptoms. Grief is much less predictable, both in my experience and from what I have observed in my practice. Grief is how we respond to and attempt to cope with losses in our life. You can develop trauma symptoms from a loss and also start the grieving process—that is where things can get confusing.

Both as a therapist and as a person who experienced loss, I operate from the school of thought that considers grief to be cumulative. What this means is that grief is a lifelong process. I will never get over losing my dad. That loss is part of me. When I get married or have children of my own, I know he will be with me in spirit, but his loss will affect me. Recently, a family member had a health scare. Although everyone and everything is fine, I felt that grief come up again. I remember my therapist calling it a gift that my grief could resurface so I could process it. As much as I want to be annoyed by his acknowledgment, I know he was correct. Many therapists and people who have been to therapy are familiar with the phrase "the way forward is through," which basically means that working through one's difficult emotions in life is better than avoiding them or bypassing them. Grief is not a single, isolated event but an ongoing journey. Additional losses or reminders of existing losses can stimulate my grief anew, and each time, the most therapeutic thing I can do is embrace the grief and move through it.

When a patient who is dealing with a trauma response is triggered, I would not typically call it a gift. I would not call it cumulative. In fact, the proof of successful trauma treatment is that triggers are less severe over time or gone completely. Additional traumatic events stacked on previous ones can make trauma symptoms more severe. I am not sure that the same thing always happens with grief. That might be true for some people, particularly if the losses occur close together. It was my experience, when my grandfather passed away, that I was better prepared to grieve the loss because I had grieved before. I know the same is true for many of my loved ones and patients who process multiple losses. On the other hand, multiple trauma responses, when stacked on one another, can leave survivors feeling less resilient and more prone to severe symptoms. These are just some of the ways that trauma and grief are different.

Just because there are some similarities between trauma and grief, that does not mean there are not important differences that warrant them being two separate constructs. In his book *The End of Trauma*, Dr. George Bonanno argues that PTSD is not as prevalent as we typically think.[1] By studying 9/11 survivors,

Dr. Bonanno reveals that many symptoms often attributed to PTSD are actually part of a natural coping process. People adapt to adversity through flexible coping strategies. While everyone possesses these strategies to varying degrees, Dr. Bonanno writes that what we sometimes think is trauma is actually just us dealing with the challenges and suffering that are part of everyone's life. After my father passed on, I had sleep problems. When I experienced panic attacks, I remember dissociating from my body. These symptoms were particularly severe in the days following his death. Disordered sleep and dissociation are symptoms of PTSD. Is it fair to say that these were trauma symptoms, or was this my nervous system's way of coping with a tragic and unexpected loss?

When people say everyone has trauma, sometimes what I think they mean is that everyone has grief. Everyone experiences loss, and everyone has to deal with it. It's an inevitable aspect of life. The loss could be the loss of a parent, as it was for me; the loss of a relationship with the person you thought you would marry; the loss of the life you thought you were going to have until you realized that destiny had other plans for you. It could be the loss of that dream job you always wanted but eventually needed to let go. It could be the loss of a pet. You may or may not develop trauma responses to these losses, but you will grieve.

I wanted to end this chapter by sharing a quote that I find particularly poignant and helpful if you are dealing with grief. The relevance and applicability of this quote to the grieving process is yet another example of how grief is different from trauma, as the words of Dietrich Bonhoeffer are not appropriate to a trauma survivor. Anyone who has had to grieve the loss of a loved one knows the special meaning his words carry.

Psychobabble

There is nothing that can replace the absence of someone dear to us, and one should not even attempt to do so. One must simply hold out and endure it. At first that sounds very hard, but at the same time it is also a great comfort. For to the extent the emptiness truly remains unfilled one remains connected to the other person through it. It is wrong to say that God fills the emptiness. God in no way fills it but much more leaves it precisely unfilled and thus helps us preserve—even in pain—the authentic relationship. Furthermore, the more beautiful and full the remembrances, the more difficult the separation. But gratitude transforms the torment of memory into silent joy. One bears what was lovely in the past not as a thorn but as a precious gift deep within, a hidden treasure of which one can always be certain.[2]

---

3 THINGS TO REMEMBER ABOUT MYTH #21: "TRAUMA IS THE SAME THING AS GRIEF"

1. Grief is the processing of a loss, while a trauma response is your mind's attempt to prevent a tragic event from happening again.

2. While trauma and grief share some similarities, they also have very important differences.

3. You do not have to lose a loved one for your grief to be valid and real.

Myth #22: "Disciplining Your Child Will Cause Trauma"

One of the fascinating consequences of the rise of mental health awareness is that many parents are particularly concerned about inadvertently traumatizing their children. Some mistakenly assume that avoiding all risk of trauma is a recipe for successful parenting. While I certainly endorse being aware of what trauma is and trying to prevent it, avoiding anything that can potentially cause a trauma response is literally impossible. We know that it's impossible based on what we know about trauma and how it works. For one thing, enforcing structure in the form of expectations and inflicting some unpleasant emotions are necessary for adequate parenting. Permissive parenting is just as risky as parenting in a way that attempts to eliminate unpleasant emotions. Experiencing unpleasant emotions is not the same thing as experiencing a trauma response.

Additionally, there is confusion largely stemming from the

fact that trauma responses are subjective. As we have seen, two people can get into the same car accident, and one will develop PTSD and one will not. Furthermore, two people with PTSD can display very different symptoms from each other: One person will avoid thinking or talking about the traumatic event, while the other will ruminate and hyperfixate on the traumatic event. People learn this about trauma and naturally assume that since trauma is subjective, any mistake they make by overdoing discipline with their children is a recipe for trauma.

Let me put your mind at ease, whether you are a parent or you have a parent. Everyone talks about their parents in therapy. Everyone processes the things that their parents did imperfectly. I have had patients who survived the most vile and horrific abuse from their parents, and I have had patients who experienced only normative conflict and disagreements with their parents. Everyone still talks about their parents. If your parents raised you in an authoritative household, you might resent them for not letting you enjoy your youth and not giving you more agency and freedom. If your parents were permissive and never punished you, you might resent them for not instilling a sense of self-control and discipline. Every parenting strategy has a downside, and those downsides will be discussed in therapy.

Real harms can arise when people are too extreme in their approaches. I am deeply skeptical of any parent who does not believe in disciplining their child. It's been my observation that these people typically think that their children are inherently good because they believe that people are inherently good. You hear them say things like "All we need is love" and blaming trauma, bad parenting, or systemic influences for any bad behavior. While some behavior may be traceable to a particular event or systemic factor, I always have the same question for these parents: Have you ever spent time in a preschool or day care? These children, ranging from two to five years old, are some of the most violent creatures on the planet. They kick, bite, steal, and scream. Some of them are sophisticated enough to throw a temper tantrum to get what they want, not just from other children, but also from the adults who look after them. Think about how wild that is: Young children have the capacity to be emotionally manipulative. They're not very sophisticated about it, but it's manipulative behavior nonetheless. It's the job of the adults in a child's life to properly socialize the child. Proper socialization often requires disciplinary action by the caregiver. Let me be clear, I am not advocating for physical discipline; I'm talking about discipline in the broadest sense possible, sometimes referred to as consequences or some sort of regulation. Whatever you call it, it is essential to the process of raising adaptive children.

I am also deeply skeptical of any parent who is overly controlling and overdisciplines their child. Parenting experts don't agree on everything, but one thing they do agree on is that your child will eventually attempt something called individuation. Individuation refers to the process of children distinguishing themselves from their parents and family of origin. When this happens, they develop a sense of self while maintaining healthy emotional connections with their family members. This can look like rebelling during the teenage years. Parents sometimes control their children by making things so comfortable that their children never want to move out. Whether you use the carrot or the stick, you're still trying to control them. Children who never individuate can struggle with developing a clear sense of self, leading to difficulties in maintaining healthy adult relationships and a sense of autonomy. I share this to point out that trauma is not the only way to mess up your child's mental health.

I find time and time again that parents benefit from three key reminders. First, balance and flexibility are key to any parenting approach. Even if you are a fervent believer in authoritative parenting, there will be times when a different approach might be more strategic. Second, socialization is not just about how you discipline children, although that is an important consideration. It's also about how you repair your relationship with them when someone makes mistakes. It's okay to make mistakes. They are inevitable. Third, embrace the cyclical nature of parent-child relationships. It's normal for people to cycle between harmony, conflict, and repair.

The best piece of therapeutic insight I can share with you, particularly if you are a parent, is this: Do not aim for perfection. Stop following all the parenting experts on social media. In fact, stop thinking therapists have all the answers, including me! Therapists are trained in fixing mental health concerns. I do not know when we became the wise sages with all the answers on the parent-child relationship, which is not only a human experience that has been going on for all of history and prehistory, but also an animal experience. All those parents managed just fine before Freud, and you will, too. Remember the saying often attributed to Donald Winnicott: The good enough parent is a parent that always fails. A good parent is not perfect, but they are *good enough*. Even though your failures and mistakes may give your child grist for the mill in therapy, you are not 100 percent responsible for their mental health outcomes, just as your parents are not 100 percent responsible for yours.

3 THINGS TO REMEMBER ABOUT MYTH #22: "DISCIPLINING YOUR CHILD WILL CAUSE TRAUMA"

1. Just because trauma is subjective, that does not mean that any discipline will traumatize your child.

2. Children are not 100 percent "good" or "bad," and they need consequences for certain behavior so they can be socialized properly.

3. In parenting, aim to be *good enough*, not perfect.

Myth #23: "Your Trauma Made You an Empath"

When Victoria came to see me, she let me know she was an empath. *Empath* is a term derived from the word *empathy*, and it describes someone who is highly sensitive to the emotions of others. They constantly feel what others are feeling. People sometimes use the term *empath* to imply that a person is sensitive, intuitive, and compassionate and has difficulties setting boundaries with other people. Victoria came to see me for therapy because her empathy was wearing her out. Her working theory was that her empathy was making her depressed because she could not turn it off. At the end of the day, she felt like a shell of a human being who had spent all her energy on others, feeling their feelings and acting accordingly.

Victoria's story is similar to many others I've encountered in my practice. Her parents were wildly emotionally immature. They were self-centered, expected their children to be adults from a young age, and could not take responsibility for their mistakes. They were also physically abusive at times. Victoria's understanding was that her parents would lash out physically when they became emotionally overwhelmed. They weren't sadists or psychopathic, but they would resort to hitting their children when they reached a boiling point.

It became clear to me, as I got to know Victoria, that she had developed at a very young age the ability to pick up on what her parents were feeling. That makes sense. If she could discern what they were feeling and stay proactively aware, she could conduct herself in a way that would help keep their emotions and behavior predictable. To achieve a sense of stability and safety, Victoria would instinctively monitor her parents' emotions to stay safe. If one of them signaled that they could be volatile, she knew to tiptoe around them. If one of them got angry, she could escape to her room.

Many people, of all genders and backgrounds, have the experience of wanting to accommodate the emotions of others. For some of these people, this desire can be temperamental. Personality researchers have conceptualized a trait called agreeableness. People who are highly agreeable tend to be compassionate, cooperative, trusting, honest, and deferential. They can be highly empathic in the sense that they feel the feelings of others and are easily moved to pity. Agreeableness is on a spectrum, so some people are highly agreeable, while others are highly disagreeable. Disagreeable people are competitive, blunt, and highly independent. They are less concerned with others' feelings and more concerned with objective truth and justice. They have no problem intimidating others to get their way. Most people are in the middle of this continuum.

Sometimes, I observe that when people use the word *empath* to describe themselves, they mean they likely score very high on the trait of agreeableness. This is particularly true when people take *empath* to mean the person has difficulties setting boundaries with others. Sometimes referred to as "people pleasers," as we've discussed earlier, such people can have a difficult time putting up guardrails to protect themselves from those who might take advantage of them. Empaths typically cite an understanding of other people's emotional motivations, while people pleasers may find conflict draining. Both tendencies are subtraits of agreeableness. Disagreeable people sometimes report finding conflict to be invigorating. It's worth noting that being disagreeable is not necessarily a bad thing. In fact, agreeable empaths and people pleasers can benefit from therapy to learn how to be more disagreeable so they can live a more fulfilled life.

It's possible that Victoria was wired to have an agreeable temperament, but I do not believe that was the main source of her empathic nature, which left her feeling drained. I think that her constant need to monitor and accommodate other people's emotions stemmed from her childhood abuse. I do not think that it's fair or accurate to say trauma made her an empath. I think the experiences of her childhood left her hypervigilant. Hypervigilance is commonly seen in PTSD. It is a state of heightened alertness to potential threats in the environment. One parallel could be a veteran who has come back from war and sees danger lurking around every corner. Being on high alert like that makes sense when you are in a war zone. When you transition back to being a civilian, it does not make as much sense.

Arguably, Victoria grew up in something like a war zone. Hypervigilance keeps soldiers safe in battle, just as it kept Victoria safe when she was a child. When a soldier comes home from war, if that hypervigilant pattern continues, it becomes what therapists call maladaptive: it is a behavior or way of thinking that does not provide adequate functioning in an environment or situation. It would not be advisable for a soldier to stop being hypervigilant in battle, just as it would not have been therapeutic for Victoria to stop emotionally monitoring everyone when she was a child under the care of abusive parents. But after the war, when Victoria had grown up, she was still being hypervigilant, which was leading her to feel burned-out and depressed.

That is what makes something disordered: that it's no longer adaptive. When a pattern or tendency is no longer helpful, it's maladaptive. When people describe themselves as empaths in the context of therapy, they are not usually describing a supernatural ability to feel what others are feeling and know what others are up to based on those feelings. Instead, these people are often describing their struggle to stop emotional monitoring. This can be a mental health concern. Emotional monitoring is possibly hypervigilance resulting from trauma but could be extreme agreeableness in the form of people-pleasing as well. Remember, pleasing people can mean a lot of things, depending on the person. For Victoria, people-pleasing meant being so cooperative, compassionate, and polite that she would not go against other people's preferences, even when it would be advantageous to do so.

My general issue with the term *empath* is that it seems to be used predominantly in spiritual communities, by self-help gurus, and on the internet, where people wear the label like a badge of honor. They are often not considering the very real possibility that their empathic compulsion is not a personality trait, gift, or skill that they intentionally developed over time. They are often not seeing the potential disordered behavior of their empathic nature, which can cause real mental health consequences when left unchecked over time. The empath identity then becomes a barrier to healing. For example, instead of healing their trauma and living a more adaptive life, such individuals might make the symptoms a part of who they are, so they are not invested in healing. Nobody should go through mental health treatment or any sort of healing journey they are not ready for; but I do take issue with the way the term *empath* can encourage people to avoid doing the work to get better. That is not the promise of the mental health field—or of most spiritual communities, for that matter.

Some people may have powerful empathic abilities. I do not stand as an authority on whether or not those people exist or what the underlying psychological or neurological or spiritual mechanisms may be. I do know that lots of people are living their lives, identifying as empaths, and they are suffering. If you are one of them, and a little therapy can alleviate your suffering, then I think it's worth recognizing that your trauma may not have made you an empath. It may have left you hypervigilant and overly attuned to the emotional needs of others.

> **3 THINGS TO REMEMBER ABOUT MYTH #23: "YOUR TRAUMA MADE YOU AN EMPATH"**
>
> 1. There is a difference between having empathy and being an empath.
>
> 2. There is a difference between being an empath, being hypervigilant, and having an agreeable personality.
>
> 3. The romanticization of being an empath can be a barrier to healing trauma.

⊗ Myth #24: "Questioning Trauma Discourse Harms Survivors"

The truth is that the mental health field has a dirty little secret. Memories are highly suggestible, and there are documented cases of people developing memories and constructing events that did not actually happen. I first learned about this phenomenon in a book called *Mistakes Were Made (but Not by Me)*.[1] The authors, Carol Tavris and Elliot Aronson, recount how certain therapeutic techniques can create memories that patients believe are real, even if they are completely made-up. Therapists who inadvertently implant false memories may justify their actions by believing they are uncovering repressed traumas. Patients who develop false memories of trauma can suffer real psychological harm. They may experience distress, strained family relationships, and even legal battles based on these false memories. One colleague told me that he knows of patients who developed personality disorders based on improperly conducted psychoanalysis in which the therapists were searching for trauma, when in fact there was none.

The good news is that it is very easy to avoid implanting false memories in patients. The bad news, from what I can tell, is that these guardrails are not often used on social media. If I am being honest, I never aspired to become the therapist who criticizes trauma discourse. I started doing so because I am aware of these risks and was shocked that many in my field were making social media videos about trauma with no consideration for the possibility that people's memories would be impacted. Even if you do not believe that false memories can be implanted, you have to consider that the meaning we make about our memories can be influenced by our therapists. When these therapists make vague and viral videos with messages like "Everyone's personality is just a trauma response" and "If you don't like to ask for help, that's from trauma," I have to question their motivations—or, at the very least, their competence.

When I first started publicly commenting that not everything can be explained by trauma, many of my colleagues agreed with me. At the same time, I received a particularly consistent thread of criticism. The criticism was this: Asking hard questions about trauma actually harms survivors, while besmirching the profession as a whole. People are concerned about this possibility because, historically, survivors of trauma often have not been believed when they asked for help or disclosed their abuse. Sometimes, trauma survivors minimize the scope of what's happened to them to the point where they are not able to admit to themselves—let alone their therapists—that anything bad happened. I have thought long and hard about this criticism. I have read additional books covering theories and conceptions about trauma that contradict my own. I've consulted with colleagues and trauma professionals about what they think. I want to address those concerns now.

One concern some people have is that by talking frankly about misuse of the concept of trauma, some survivors may question whether or not their trauma is real. I have never encountered a patient who was able to identify and process a trauma, and then—because of a few words from a random therapist on the internet—suppressed, forgot, or doubted everything that happened. I have never come across such a case in any outpatient setting I have worked in or in any case study I have read. Yes, people minimize their painful and traumatic memories. But I have never known a case of a person being aware that they have trauma and then claiming that the conversations I have outlined about trauma caused them to doubt that their trauma was real.

I have asked several trusted colleagues whether they thought this was happening to patients in treatment who encountered my message. Not a single colleague was concerned. I even reached out to trauma specialists I didn't know very well to see what they thought. The general takeaway from all my consultations was that people who struggle with black-and-white thinking, sometimes known as binary thinking, may hear criticisms about trauma discourse and interpret them to mean that trauma isn't important, trauma isn't real, or "your trauma didn't happen to you." In other words, every professional I have consulted agrees that my message is important to put into public discourse and that it's not actually harming anyone. If it is causing distress, it is distress that is easily remedied by consulting a licensed professional.

One colleague was able to share about a patient she treats who has a hard time letting themselves remember their trauma; this conversation focused on working with dissociative amnesia in trauma treatment. My colleague's sense was that if she had a patient whose media consumption was triggering dissociative amnesic episodes, she would direct the patient to stop consuming certain kinds of content until treatment had progressed. She also wondered whether people take my message to mean they experience a feeling of shock and disbelief that something happened to them, which is markedly different from not being able to remember the trauma.

My concerns about the misuse of the term *trauma* are shared by my senior colleagues in the field. They are echoed by many practitioners and researchers. Many people agree with me, and many people do not. This is a debate my field is having, and anyone who wishes to learn about psychology and mental health will likely encounter this debate. When I spoke to Matthias Barker, the CEO of the Trauma Institute, he told me he defines any psychogenic event that leads to an ongoing maladaptive response as a trauma.[2] I countered this definition with an example. If someone grew up being the class clown and was having a hard time adjusting to being a young adult after college because he could no longer be the jokester, then he is dealing with an ongoing maladaptive pattern. While he could have developed this personality in response to a trauma, it is highly likely that the appropriate therapy would focus on a life transition. Matthias disagreed. Matthias felt that something must have happened to him to make him want to be the jokester, and it was our job, as trauma-informed therapists, to find out what happened so that therapy can be curative.

I don't think Matthias is a bad therapist. In fact, I think he's a good one. I do not think he is causing anyone harm. In fact, I think he's helping a ton of people with his content. It's worth pointing out that, at the time of our interview, he had never read *Mistakes Were Made (but Not by Me)*. I believe he would be an even better therapist if he learned about the potential to instill false memories. I know that I am a better therapist for having spoken to him, and I am sure I would be better if I took courses or read books that Matthias recommends. Many professionals have differing opinions, and that's okay. It's important for me, for him, and for other therapists to voice their concerns about mental health–related discourse, so we can all be better. It's important that we all participate in this conversation if we have something to say. For example, our conversation was super interesting and productive, but conversations do not need to take place on a podcast to meaningfully impact the field. They can occur between clinicians or between students who are learning all that they can to be the best they can be.

I want to leave you with a few more thoughts about people who claim we cannot have conversations about trauma because the discourse is harmful. My interpretation is threefold. First, the people who make this claim may be in a place, mentally, where they cannot handle learning about different debates in the field. They should exercise caution when doing research on their own, especially on social media, and they should seek support from a qualified professional. Second, people who make this claim disagree with my philosophical stances on trauma. They are allowed to disagree, but they must push back against my argument itself. They should not simply cite "harm" without addressing any of my concerns.

Finally, and perhaps most tragically, some who seek to quash nuanced discourse about trauma-related topics may be possessed by something called pathological compassion. Pathological compassion, often referred to as toxic empathy, manifests as an excessive and rigid form of empathy in which an individual demonstrates care and concern for others to the point of harm. This concept is related to the archetype of the *devouring mother*, a term rooted in Jungian psychology that describes caregivers who smother and overwhelm their children, infantilizing them and stifling their progress and sense of agency in the process. These people are welcome to criticize my concerns about trauma and related mental health discourse. At the same time, their personal motivations should be considered as we decide what weight to give their criticisms.

Remember, when treating trauma, one of the biggest mistakes a therapist can make is to push a patient to process things too quickly. But it's also a big mistake to treat a patient as though they're more fragile than they actually are.

> **3 THINGS TO REMEMBER ABOUT MYTH #24: "QUESTIONING TRAUMA DISCOURSE HARMS SURVIVORS"**
>
> 1. There are real risks to psychotherapy when it's improperly conducted.
>
> 2. It's important to talk about these risks, even if doing so causes unpleasant feelings or complications with ongoing treatment.
>
> 3. Questioning trauma discourse helps both survivors and the mental health field.

Part V

Social Schisms: Common Myths About Mental Health and Society

Myth #25: "Your Mental Illness Is a Systemic Problem"

Individual responsibility and systemic change are not at odds with each other when it comes to improving mental health. Individual responsibility is the accountability of every person to make actions and choices and live with those consequences. Systemic change refers to the transformation of societal structures, policies, and norms within a society. Some of you might read that and think, *makes perfect sense to me*. Others may have an unpleasant emotional reaction. On my social media, I have created posts on this topic, and I have always found it curious how political this topic gets for people. While this chapter may be interpreted as political, I want to be clear that's not my intention. I have done the best I can to remain strictly in the clinical and philosophical domain. It's important for you to understand that the psychological field is deeply divided about whether mental health problems are inherently systemic. My hope is that you will be a better advocate for your stance on this issue by considering the nuances and perspectives on all sides of the debate.

Cathy was a single mom who was at her wits' end. She was struggling to make ends meet for her children, and the struggle was causing her to lose sleep and feel depressed. She was completely burned-out. After assessing Cathy, I told her that anyone would be feeling stressed and depressed in her circumstances. It seemed to me that her depression and anxiety were normal responses to really tough circumstances. If she had more money or more support, she would likely be less stressed. Just hearing that there was nothing wrong with her mind was incredibly therapeutic for Cathy. She was under the impression that something was fundamentally flawed about her because she was feeling burned-out. By explaining the biological and psychological mechanisms of burnout, I was able to relieve some of the burden she was carrying. Ultimately, she decided to go on medication to give her the extra kick she needed to get financially stable. Once her finances were normalized, she experienced massive symptom relief and was able to go off medication.

When Devon came to see me, I was working at a clinic that accepts patients on Medicaid. Devon was on the verge of homelessness. I referred him to a social worker at my clinic who was able to help him find housing for his family. Housing was—miraculously—secured very promptly, but Devon's symptoms worsened. He was dealing with grief and PTSD from witnessing his family member die in a car accident. Devon was distraught because he had hoped that all his problems would get better when he received housing, but that didn't happen. I explained that grief takes time, and I encouraged him to consider trauma therapy, either with me or with a trauma specialist at the clinic. Devon wasn't ready to talk about what happened and refused a medication consultation. He showed up to sessions for therapy but did not engage. Eventually, he resorted to virtual sessions because he was too anxious to leave the house. My supervisor cautioned me not to push him, so I didn't. I was patient, validating, and accepting of him and the situation he found himself in. He was so resistant to even gentle interventions that he asked to see another therapist, whom he also quickly fired. The other therapist advised me to not take this personally. It was her assessment that Devon simply wasn't ready, and it was not our job to make him ready. He was going to continue to engage in behaviors that would make his symptoms worse until he was ready to get help to stop them.

What do these stories have to do with individual responsibility and systemic responsibility when it comes to progress in therapy? Each story highlights how individuality and collective responsibility are two sides of the same coin—not separate concepts. In conversations about mental health, many people, including therapists, will feel strongly about whether to prioritize individual agency or systems thinking. I want to go on record as saying that you need to integrate these two perspectives to help someone therapeutically—or even to understand your own problems.

One way to understand how to balance these perspectives is through the concept of locus of control, or LOC. LOC is about the extent to which an individual believes they have the power to control what happens in their life. If they feel like they have a lot of influence over the outcomes of their life, they have a high internal LOC. Many studies find that an internal LOC is associated with better mental health outcomes.[1] People with an external LOC believe that their lives are controlled by external factors. People with a high external LOC are more likely to experience depression and more likely to be negatively impacted by stress. Additionally, those with an external LOC who have depression tend to have worse mental health symptoms than those who have a high internal LOC. A thorough reading of the literature makes it clear that when it comes to mental health, leaning toward an internal LOC predicts better outcomes.

At the end of the day, any therapist who validates only an external LOC may be encouraging a victim mindset that could make mental health symptoms worse. At the same time, therapists who encourage only an internal LOC may inadvertently shame their patients and, ironically, decrease a sense of agency. The approach depends on how ready the patient is to make a change. Considering all the factors, a willingness to change and an openness to do "the work" really make a big difference in therapeutic outcomes.

If I had only assured Cathy that it wasn't her fault about her mental health situation, that would not have been enough. She needed comfort, validation, and a weight taken off her shoulders, but she also needed motivation, resolve, and resilience. Although her situation might not have been her fault, it was her responsibility to do something about it. She chose to get what she needed through medication, but she could have taken action in other ways. Medication is not the only solution for people who find themselves cornered by life's circumstances. If I hadn't encouraged an internal LOC, I would have run the risk of encouraging a victim mindset.

If Devon had been less resistant to therapy, or if I or the other practitioner had figured out an approach to Devon that motivated him, he would have started to get better. Systemic support in the form of housing likely made his problems worse, because he was finally able to slow down and feel the depth of his grief and trauma. When we have space to slow down, we have space to heal; but, unfortunately, healing often begins with feeling the pain and emotions that we have been avoiding. If I had simply validated Devon's frustrations that finding housing didn't alleviate his other problems, he might have stayed in therapy longer, but I am not sure whether he would have gotten better. He needed to process his grief and trauma. Sometimes, I think about Devon. Sometimes, I view his case as one in which I made many mistakes. Perhaps I should have let him signal that he was ready to do something about his circumstances? Maybe I wasn't sensitive enough to how hard his circumstances were to contend with?

There is no clear answer here. This is not an either-or decision. The main takeaway is that when you encounter arguments about the role of systemic change versus individual responsibility in mental health, be wary of how narrow-minded the people making these arguments might be.

---

3 THINGS TO REMEMBER ABOUT MYTH #25: "YOUR MENTAL ILLNESS IS A SYSTEMIC PROBLEM"

1. Therapists who encourage only an external locus of control may be ignoring evidence-based practices and encouraging a victim mindset.

2. Therapists who encourage only an internal locus of control may inadvertently shame their patients and—ironically—decrease their sense of agency.

3. Individual responsibility and systemic considerations can and should be integrated into psychotherapy together.

⊗ Myth #26: "People Aren't Evil, They're Just Mentally Ill"

In a TEDx Talk titled "The Most Important Lesson from 83,000 Brain Scans," Dr. Daniel Amen tells a story about how a nine-year-old boy violently attacked a little girl on the baseball field.[1] The boy had been drawing pictures of himself hanging from a tree and shooting other children. It was later revealed that the boy had a cyst in his brain. When the cyst was removed, his violent impulses and thoughts went away completely. He turned back into a sweet and loving little boy. The boy was Dr. Amen's nephew. Dr. Amen points out that this was likely a Columbine or Sandy Hook waiting to happen.

Aaron Hernandez, a tight end for the New England Patriots, is infamous for murdering his friend Odin Lloyd. Hernandez was diagnosed with chronic traumatic encephalopathy (CTE), and that diagnosis is used to explain his actions.[2] Dr. Ann McKee, a neuropathologist who studies CTE, said, "We can't take the pathology and explain the behavior, but we can say collectively that individuals with CTE of this severity have difficulty with impulse control, decision-making, aggression, often emotional volatility, and rage behavior."[3] Both Dr. Amen's nephew and Aaron Hernandez are examples of chilling, yet hopeful, stories about how seemingly unexplainable and atrocious acts may have an underlying, explainable, medical cause.

Personally, I find it encouraging that when people hear about something heinous and awful on the news, they say something like "That's so sick that they did that." If a person is sick, then maybe they can be cured. It's encouraging that people want to be able to explain the awful things that human beings sometimes do to one another. These people are trying to see the best in others. When people view bad, evil, or antisocial behavior through a mental health lens, that's what they are trying to do. They believe that if the person had been raised properly or had received the right treatment, they wouldn't have done those things. People have these beliefs because there is some compelling evidence for them.

According to the Traumatic Brain Injury in Criminal Justice Project at the University of Denver Graduate School of Professional Psychology, some jails have up to 96 percent of inmates with a history of at least one traumatic brain injury, or TBI.[4] While rates of TBI vary among sites, again, some view that statistic with a certain degree of hope. Outside of brain cysts and complex TBIs, we have data showing that people with bipolar disorder or a schizophrenia-related disorder are more likely to end up in jail. One study found that people with ADHD are more likely to end up in prison[5]—which makes sense, because if you have poor impulse control, you are more likely to do something without thinking that might get you in trouble.

When someone commits a crime, I agree they deserve the best representation imaginable. If a mental health argument will help someone's case, lawyers should make that argument. If mental health is a factor to consider in the outcome of a trial, it should definitely be taken into account. But does the tendency to explain away sins, mistakes, and crimes against society by pointing to mental illness end up confusing and obscuring the difference between behavior we deem bad and mental illness itself? In other words, is there perhaps an inflation of the idea that mental illness and bad behavior are correlated because lawyers will lean on the mental health argument if they can? If that's true, then as a mental health culture, we need to be sure not to get seduced by the psychobabble around comparing and contrasting mental illness and acts we collectively wish to punish as a society.

One major problem with the myth that people are not bad, just mentally ill, is that it implies that people with a mental illness are more likely to commit crimes, commit heinous acts, or get into trouble. This is not just false—it is illogical. First of all, all dogs are mammals, but that doesn't mean all mammals are dogs. Just because those who are in jail happen to have higher rates of mental illness or TBIs, that doesn't mean those with mental illness or TBIs are more likely to commit crimes. In fact, a large body of data shows that people with mental illness are much more likely to be victims of violent crime than the perpetrators of it.[6] In one study looking at violence and schizophrenia, it was shown that substance use was a better predictor than just having schizophrenia.[7] In fact, alcohol is a key factor in most violent crime, regardless of your mental health status.[8]

The idea that we can explain away bad behavior through mental health is alluring because we don't like to consider that we are all capable of terrible things. If someone hurts us physically, it's somewhat comforting to think they have something wrong with their minds or brains. If someone hurts our feelings, it's reassuring to consider that their agitation stemmed from a childhood wound or being overdue for an adjustment with their medication. It's terrifying to believe that someone would hurt us soberly, consciously, and intentionally. That would mean people you trust—people you love—might be capable of a similar transgression. It's even more intimidating to consider that you might be capable of doing things you believe are wrong.

There are many perspectives about whether or not people are naturally good or bad. I believe that we all have capacity for both good and evil. I am particularly fond of Carl Jung's analysis, that accepting the fact that you *are* capable of absolutely horrible things is a mark of maturity. His argument is that if you are aware of your capacity for evil, then you can keep an eye on it and conduct yourself in a good or moral fashion. Jung believed that it is not a lack of capacity for bad behavior that makes someone good; the people who can do bad things but choose not to are the ones who are truly good. Jung thought that people who delude themselves into thinking that they can never do anything that bad are the people who end up committing the most atrocious acts. He also thought that it was unfair to the people who consciously choose good over evil to label people who are incapable of doing bad things as the most moral, because they don't have a choice in the matter.

I had a mentor tell me that in order to become truly masterful in the art and science of psychology, you need to think about deep and dark questions. You need to consider whether or not each and every person has the capacity to do bad things. In my opinion, these sorts of questions quickly leave the realm of psychology and touch on questions of philosophy and even theology. In philosophy, as in psychology, it's vital to define your terms. I do not have a deep or concise definition of bad or evil that I can offer you to contextualize the ideas presented in this chapter. I do not think I need one. If your thinking is that good and evil are totally subjective and do not exist, then you don't agree with the myth by default. If evil doesn't exist, then comparing mental illness to evil is a moot point. Furthermore, I cannot imagine a working definition of evil that would conflict with the larger point of this chapter: While mental and physical health might explain some behavior we can classify as bad, it simply cannot explain all of it. To try to convince you otherwise would make me feel like I was trying to sell you a story rather than telling you the truth.

---

3 THINGS TO REMEMBER ABOUT MYTH #26: "PEOPLE AREN'T EVIL, THEY'RE JUST MENTALLY ILL"

1. There is some bad, evil, or antisocial behavior that can be explained by undiagnosed illness, which is likely more biological than mental in nature.

2. Be careful of further stigmatizing mental illness by associating criminality and mental illness.

3. Reconsider whether or not the best way to be a good person is to believe you are incapable of being bad.

Myth #27: "Mental Health Education Is Always Beneficial"

My patient AJ had been through years of therapy and was relatively low-functioning. At the age of thirty, he didn't have a job and lived at home with his family. He had spent years thinking about his problems and had several therapists who did extensive psychoanalytical work with him. From what I could tell, they helped him talk about his problems but never provided any feedback, tools, or interventions, just more processing. The result was that AJ was very good at talking about his problems and knew how to conduct a cogent self-analysis. At the same time, he seemed surprised when I offered to help him think about solutions to his problems. AJ's expectation of therapy was that he could only talk about his issues.

One session, AJ told me that he wanted me, his therapist, to be similar to his bartender—someone who listened but didn't really try to fix anything. I wish AJ's previous therapists had looked at the whole picture. I wish they had looked into medication, sleep hygiene, and something like dialectical behavior therapy so AJ could be armed with tools to make changes, not just talk about problems. I don't really blame his previous therapists, though. AJ always had a colorful and dramatic story about why he left each one. Maybe they just weren't a good fit. Maybe something deeper was going on. A big part of our work together was agreeing on what therapy was for and how to get the most out of it. Personally and professionally, I was uncomfortable being labeled as a bartender, even metaphorically.

    I believe that AJ's previous therapists failed him. In my clinical training, I was shocked to learn that more mental health education and intervention does not always lead to better mental health outcomes. In fact, often it can harm your mental health. This makes sense if you think about it. Constantly thinking about your problems all day can lead to rumination, obsession, and more anxiety. Rumination is often a symptom of depression. Learning about psychology may be intellectually stimulating, but that does not mean you are doing the work necessary to grow, heal, and improve your mental health. Some practitioners refer to this as intellectualizing, where you think about and reason through an issue instead of feeling uncomfortable emotions. Additionally, just because you have insight into the causes of your problems, that does not mean you have applied those insights to any potential solutions. More talking about your problems is not always what is needed.

    Most therapists learn this their first year of grad school. It can be tempting to want to educate your patients about all the cool stuff you have learned. I know I was a bit like this with my first patients. I was so excited to explain things and teach them about their mind and brain. I quickly learned that was not always what was needed. Interestingly, as mental health has become less stigmatized, people hope to apply insights from the mental health field to school, work, child-rearing, and more. Unfortunately, I have noticed a trend where people mistakenly assume that more mental health education is better because mental health can apply to everything.

Because therapy is time-consuming and costly, and resources are limited, it's appealing to take pieces of psychotherapy and try to water them down to benefit many people in the population. This has been true when it comes to adolescent mental health in the United States. In November 2023, Dr. Darby Saxbe of the University of Southern California penned an op-ed called "This Is Not the Way to Help Depressed Teenagers."[1] Dr. Saxbe reviewed studies showing that different initiatives to improve teenage mental health were making mental health symptoms worse. She points to large-scale and light-touch interventions in the mental health crisis following COVID-19, which seemed appealing because they had the potential to help many people. Social emotional learning workshops, mindfulness classes, sharing circles, and various seminars have been leveraged to try to help those in need improve their mental health. Teenagers are often resistant to attending therapy, so many well-intentioned individuals hoped that psychotherapy-adjacent interventions would help. They were wrong. She points out that if you really wanted to improve teenage mental health, you could just start class later in the day and allow teenagers to get more sleep. That recommendation isn't as appealing as a takeaway from a cutting-edge mindfulness seminar. Implementing a later start time would also require logistic adjustments, such as changes to bus schedules and parents' work schedules, making it less desirable.

In February 2024, Abigail Shrier's book *Bad Therapy: Why the Kids Aren't Growing Up* was published.[2] The author investigates potential reasons why child and adolescent mental health has never been worse even though we, as a society, have never paid more attention to it or invested more money into it than we do today. One of her main points is that talking about your problems all the time can make you feel worse. Some people need to learn how to talk about their problems to get better, but there are lots of other ways to improve your mental health that have nothing to do with therapy.

At first I thought that these failures of society-wide mental health interventions were a phenomenon exclusive to the post-COVID era. It made sense to me that as mental health stigma decreased, efforts to improve mental health would increase, and things would get improperly applied in the shuffle. I am no longer sure that is a good explanation. In the 1990s, trigger warnings were introduced on feminist message forums to help readers prepare for or avoid material that might trigger their PTSD or trauma symptoms. Over time, trigger warnings crept into academia and the media landscape. Trigger warnings had good intentions. When someone with PTSD is reminded of their traumatic experience, this trigger can have severe effects. Survivors can become disassociated from their bodies or become extremely dysregulated and emotional. It can last hours or even days without relief. Surely, including these would be supportive and helpful to all those who are dealing with trauma symptoms, right?

Maybe trigger warnings achieved their intended aim when they were first introduced and utilized on internet message boards in the 1990s, but times have changed. It's important to note that trigger warnings are different from content warnings. A content warning might appear before a television episode to let you know there is a depiction of violence or foul language. Today, trigger warnings are not helpful for survivors processing their trauma; nor do they serve to help people better engage with potentially distressing material. Trigger warnings have become more about emotional comfort than preventing a potential dissociative episode. If trigger warnings are aimed at ensuring a profound sense of psychological comfort, they fail at their job. Furthermore, if you are healing from a trauma, isn't it better to focus on therapy and desensitize yourself to the triggers so you can watch that movie, read that book, or participate in that discussion that had a trigger warning?

A recent meta-analysis found trigger warnings do not work.[3] Remember, a meta-analysis is a study of a group of studies on the same topic. In this meta-analysis, most studies found that trigger warnings had no impact or even made negative emotional responses worse, not better. Results were mixed as to whether or not trigger warnings encouraged people to avoid the material. For example, if a person saw a trigger warning about racism, it was unclear whether it would cause the person to engage with the material with caution or to avoid it altogether. Every single study reviewed concluded that trigger warnings consistently increased something called anticipatory anxiety, which occurs when someone imagines a future event bringing stress or discomfort.

Here's the thing: Despite the research on the matter, I am not sure that I am against trigger warnings. I see how it could be helpful for someone healing from PTSD to be alerted if material might trigger them into having a flashback. The unfortunate thing about these studies, by my assessment, is that they do not differentiate between the people with clinically significant mental health issues who would greatly need to avoid their triggers and the people who engage in trigger warnings because they are neurotic. Trait neuroticism is being sensitive to negative emotion. It can go up or down with therapy or life experience. What happened is that the good intentions of people wishing for trigger warnings to help people ended up creating an intervention that is ineffective at best and slightly harmful at worst. The biggest harm is perhaps the fact that survivors of trauma will not be taken seriously due to the ambiguous nature of trigger warnings and the accompanying research.

It's important to note that the irony is not lost on me that I am writing a book chock-full of mental health education for a popular audience, in which I am arguing that more is not always better when it comes to mental health education and intervention. Nonetheless, we have proof that mental health education can be harmful when improperly applied. Of course, misinformation can be harmful because it's incorrect; but information can also be harmful, when it's misapplied or misunderstood. My hope is that this chapter, just like all the others, encourages you to take a beat when you learn something new about mental health or human psychology—and helps you get more curious and thoughtful as you make decisions both in therapy and in life.

**3 THINGS TO REMEMBER ABOUT MYTH #27:
"MENTAL HEALTH EDUCATION IS ALWAYS BENEFICIAL"**

1. More processing is not always better when you can apply your insights to productive change.

2. Large-scale, light-touch mental health interventions can have effects that are the opposite of what was intended.

3. When it comes to improving mental health, good intentions and scalable interventions do not always have good outcomes.

Myth #28: "Psychotherapy Is the Only Way to Improve Your Mental Well-Being"

Lots of people think that psychotherapy is the only way to improve their mental health, but that's not true. In graduate school, I learned about the biopsychosocial model of mental health. In simple terms, the model shows that we have to consider biological, psychological, and social aspects of mental well-being. A biological aspect of mental health could be about medication, but it could also pertain to sleep, nutrition, exercise, or underlying physical illnesses. Psychological aspects of mental health could be about trauma, disordered thinking, or core beliefs that interrupt optimal functioning. Social aspects of mental health include the relationships in your life, the place you work, your family and upbringing, and even broader societal structures and paradigms. A good therapist can and should consider the biopsychosocial model in your treatment plan, but a great and ethical therapist will be honest with you and clarify that there are lots of ways and lots of people who can help improve your mental health. Mental health professionals offer just one way to do this work.

When Deborah came to see me, she was experiencing severe anxiety: "A few weeks ago, I noticed that I have these uncontrollable thoughts that something bad is going to happen." She denied having thoughts like this in her past. Deborah said that if she left home for work, she would be plagued with a fear that she had left her curling iron plugged into the outlet. She would become really preoccupied with the idea that the house would burn down. She thought about how her partner would have his headphones in and not hear the fire alarm and would be trapped inside. When I asked her if she thought the fire alarm might be louder than her partner's headphones, she cracked a painful smile. Deborah explained that she knew these thoughts were not rational. She knew fire alarms were louder than her partner's headphones, which were not noise-canceling. She knew that her curling iron had a safety switch, and she knew her house had sprinklers in case of a fire. None of that mattered. Her anxieties were constant and intrusive, and she was hoping to get a little relief.

The first thing I did was explain the biopsychosocial model of mental health to Deborah. I told her that I could be the best therapist for her, but she needed to get blood work done. I assured her that I would start treating her problems as if they were purely psychological but advised that she needed to talk to her doctor. Sure enough, my hunch was right. Deborah had extremely low levels of vitamin D and vitamin B_{12}, both of which are associated with anxiety symptoms. As it turns out, Deborah had recently switched to a vegan diet, which can make it difficult to get enough vitamin D and vitamin B_{12}.

After her doctor educated her on how to get the right nutrients and prescribed a couple of supplements, her anxiety symptoms went away completely. I'll never forget how happy Deborah was in the session when she told me, "I have never felt better!" Her smile was so big and infectious. It's worth noting, for all the vegans out there, that I am not for or against any sort of diet for your mental health, but this is a known complication of plant-based diets.

I did not treat Deborah very long. I didn't need to because the etiology—the origin—of her mental illness was not psychological. It would have been so unfortunate if I had wasted weeks of Deborah's time looking for repressed memories, screening for trauma symptoms, administering behavioral skills, or trying to conduct cognitive therapy, when that wasn't what she needed. She had a really blessed upbringing, a good relationship with her partner, and a fulfilling career. In fact, that's one of the things that led me to believe her anxiety might be biological. It came out of nowhere, and it didn't make sense. It might seem like an extreme example, but it's common for people to have nutritional deficiencies or disordered sleep patterns or to have not exercised in years and then report having anxiety or depression symptoms. My attitude is to always consider these factors when formulating a treatment plan.

When a patient is experiencing severe distress from their mental health problems, like Deborah, I still generally recommend therapy, even if the cause is not psychological. A competent therapist will be able to help you coordinate with other types of professionals if you need something beyond the "talking cure."

Many people seek out therapy for normative experiences of anxiety, depression, or stress. There is a difference between mental illness and "problems of living" that everyone experiences. There is a difference between trying to heal mental illness and trying to optimize mental wellness. In the latter case, the solution is usually about learning to effectively cope with problems of living in a way that works for the individual in question.

When someone comes to me and they're trying to figure out how to cope with problems of living, therapy can often help. For many people, it helps to talk about their problems. Lots of people don't have enough people in their lives to be open and vulnerable with, and psychotherapy is a wonderful site to experience that sort of relationship and reap the benefits of it. At the same time, I would argue that there are many ways to improve your well-being outside of psychotherapy. Something doesn't need to be clinical psychotherapy to feel therapeutic. Just as there is a difference between going to a mental health hospital and a wellness retreat center, there are going to be differences in the options available to you if what you want is to improve your general well-being.

Personally, I have been to lots and lots of psychotherapy. For me, it's seasonal; there will be months—years even—where I focus on my mental health. In other seasons of my life, therapy is not what's needed; instead, I will get a personal trainer, receive a massage, or work less. Therapy is expensive, and while it's been life-changing for me, there are other ways to optimize my well-being. Exercise always seems to help moderate my ADHD symptoms. I hold all my stress in my neck and shoulders. If I am not paying for therapy, I don't necessarily need to work as many hours to afford it. Having another free hour to myself during the week is beneficial.

It may feel daunting or confusing to start to consider ways to improve your mental health that are not psychotherapy. A great and effective way to explore different options is to talk to a therapist. Everyone is different, and every case is complex. The thing that works for me might not work for you. For example, having more free time in a week is good for my mental health; but for a patient who is unemployed or works only part-time, sometimes the best thing they can do for their mental health is to work more, not less. Some people benefit from the gym; others need to let themselves be unproductive and relax. If you don't know how to start mapping out what does or does not work for you, a therapist can help you figure it out.

I will end by telling you what I often tell my patients. Their care plan is a ship, and they are the captain. The therapist is their cocaptain. The therapist can help coordinate with the other crew members of the care team. Maybe there's a couples therapist, a psychiatrist, or another doctor of some sort. Maybe there's an acupuncturist or a pastor who's part of the equation as well. At the end of the day, as the captain, you call the shots for how the ship should run. Your therapist can help take some of that load off your plate if you need some additional assistance.

---

3 THINGS TO REMEMBER ABOUT MYTH #28: "PSYCHOTHERAPY IS THE ONLY WAY TO IMPROVE YOUR MENTAL WELL-BEING"

1. There is a difference between healing mental illness and improving mental wellness.

2. Psychotherapy is not the only way to feel better when it comes to your mental well-being.

3. A good therapist will help you get support wherever you need it, even if it's not psychotherapy.

Myth #29: "Party Animals Have Issues"

As a therapist, I was amused to learn that many people think that to be mentally healthy means you must be sober, celibate, or straight edge. Of course, there's nothing wrong with being any of these things. But just as being sober or celibate doesn't mean you are free from psychological problems, being someone who imbibes or partakes doesn't guarantee that you will develop a mental health concern. Some people who love to party are incredibly well-adjusted. And some people who keep themselves very pure have serious mental health issues.

How can you tell what is or isn't a mental health problem when it comes to substances and sex? The field solves for this issue by delineating that something is a mental health concern if there is social, relational, or occupational dysfunction. If you open the DSM-V, you will notice that it does not talk about addiction to substances, but rather substance *misuse*. If you are misusing a substance, then it may require clinical attention. Simply put, you are misusing a substance if you are unable to meet your goals, but you keep on misusing the substance anyway. For example, if someone enjoys drinking wine, but they are still able to meet all their goals, then their drinking is not an issue.

Addiction is real. Some people need to be sober, but that is not the focus of this chapter. Many people have difficulty seeing how to change their relationship to partying to make their lives more aligned with their values. People who have gray-area issues with drinking or sex do not necessarily fit the criteria for mild substance misuse disorder, but their problems still warrant therapeutic attention.

When Bobby came to see me, he was concerned about his drinking. As we started our work together, it became clear that Bobby was drinking to feel less anxious. When he was at a bar, Bobby was terrified to approach women he wanted to meet. If he was frozen by social anxiety, he would remain that way until he had a drink. It is not surprising that Bobby had developed a concern about his drinking, because he was not drinking to chase positive emotion. He was drinking to avoid negative emotion. There is an important difference.

If you indulge to chase pleasure, then you are not using your indulgences as a coping skill. When it comes to coping skills, diversity is key. There is nothing wrong with indulging in hedonistic pleasures to take the edge off a long day. There is nothing inherently detrimental about having a drink, hooking up with someone, or eating a tasty treat to move away from negative emotions. Bobby started to get in trouble when his coping skill—drinking—became the only one he relied on. You need a variety of coping skills because, inevitably, one will not work for you. The most beautiful person you know with the most perfect body does not necessarily have sex every time they need to relieve stress. Some nights it will be okay to have a drink, but sometimes it won't be the best idea. Exercise is a great coping skill, but on some days work will be too demanding for you to fit in your regular gym routine.

In addition to practicing other coping skills, Bobby also needed to shift his mindset about negative emotions. From a neurobiological perspective, pleasure and pain sort of dance with each other. In therapy, the pleasure-pain dance is one in which you slowly and voluntarily expose yourself to painful or unpleasant experiences. You do so to learn to tolerate discomfort. The more negative emotion you can tolerate, the more positive emotion you will be able to access. With Bobby, we eventually worked his way up to a homework assignment. Bobby had to approach fifty women when he was completely sober and ask for their numbers.

Bobby and I had developed good rapport before I suggested such an intimidating assignment. He eventually approached fifty people. And what happened? He got rejected. Sometimes they were nice about it. Sometimes they weren't so nice. Bobby's fears were not unfounded. They were informed by having been rejected before. Bobby's problem was that he learned to cope with his anxieties about rejection through alcohol. He had to learn the best way to build resilience to his insecurities so they had a smaller impact on whether or not he approached someone. Today, Bobby can still drink with the best of them, but he knows how to keep an eye on it. And he has a girlfriend—a woman he approached in a bar.

Not all patients' stories are like Bobby's. Other people are able to navigate their relationship to pleasure through different ways. For example, when Aaron came to see me, his therapy was not about desensitizing himself to unpleasant emotions. Aaron had to learn what he authentically enjoyed in his sex life. Aaron wanted to experiment with opening up his relationship with his boyfriend. He wanted to have sex with other people. After a while, Aaron let me know that whenever he tried to be with other people, he had erection difficulties, and if he managed to maintain an erection, he was rarely able to orgasm.

As I worked with Aaron, I noticed that he was very good at convincing himself that his feelings were wrong. Do you ever do this in sex or in life? Do you ever talk yourself out of how you're feeling? When Aaron and his partner were exclusive, he would make it wrong. He didn't feel like he was doing what gay men were *supposed* to be doing—being open. When they were open, he would feel jealousy or insecurity. He would say things like "It's not right for me to tell my partner what he can and cannot do if we're open ... after all, it's his body. I can't tell him what he can or cannot do with his body." His reframes didn't help him at all. He was experiencing significant levels of anxiety and losing sleep. A big part of my work with him was building a sense of self-esteem to own what he wanted.

This is called the craft of self-attunement. If you are a parent, attunement is your ability to be aware of and respond to your child's needs, especially when the child cannot necessarily articulate their needs themselves. Self-attunement is the ability to listen to your nervous system and discern your own needs. This is often easier said than done, because what we need and what we want may not always be aligned. Gay men, most of whom have spent at least some time in the closet, are often talented at suppressing their own needs. Not knowing what they want is a problem that plagues many people, regardless of their gender or sexuality. This problem can make navigating your relationship to pleasure confusing.

I told Aaron about two gay men with whom I am friends. One is in an open relationship, and one is not. My friend who is in an open relationship gets aroused when he sees someone touching his partner in a sensual way on the dance floor. At the very least, it fills him with delight to know that his partner is enjoying himself. That feeling of delight is sometimes called compersion—the opposite of jealousy. My other friend is in a monogamous relationship. He told me that the idea of his partner being sexual with someone else made him want to throw up.

I explained to Aaron that we can't judge either one of my friends for having relationships that work for them. They are owning what they like, not what others expect them to enjoy. They give themselves, and each other, flexibility in their needs, wants, and desires. Sometimes, my friend who is open doesn't want to share his partner. He communicates that. Sometimes, my other friend, in the sanctity and privacy of his monogamous commitment, will fantasize about other people out loud while having sex with his partner.

It's one thing to understand intellectually what you want or need. It's a completely different thing to experience asking for it. My work with Aaron reminds me that when it comes to sex and eroticism, people often are better off discerning what they like, not what others expect them to enjoy. Today, Aaron isn't totally open with his partner, but they are not monogamous either. He is practicing the craft of self-attunement and has figured out an arrangement that works for him. His relationship, his sex life, and his mental health are better for it.

Many people—including some therapists—would be quick to tell Bobby he has to stop drinking and would rush to convince Aaron he is not wired to be in an open relationship. It's my view that these judgments are sorely lacking in the curiosity that's needed to help people develop a deeper understanding of themselves. Lots of people who are struggling to admit that they have a problem with drinking will insist they need to figure out their deeper reason for doing what they do in order to solve the problem. Some benefit from acknowledging that they're not party animals but are struggling with substance misuse.

The last thing I want is for people who are struggling with recovery to take this chapter as license to delay the inevitable work needed in terms of being sober. More nuanced conversations about these topics, however, can benefit many people and mental health culture in general. Throughout history, human beings have used substances to alter their consciousness and have experimented with a variety of sexual and romantic arrangements. Researchers have found evidence of opium use in ancient Mesopotamia. The Romans imbibed alcoholic beverages during their feasts and Bacchanalia. The Inca used coca leaves, the source of cocaine, to enhance performance and in religious ceremonies. Sex and substances are not new, nor are humans likely to stop enjoying them anytime soon. It is the job of the therapist to make sure that regardless of how you navigate these areas of your life, you are also meeting your goals and avoiding any unnecessary dysfunction.

**3 THINGS TO REMEMBER ABOUT MYTH #29:
"PARTY ANIMALS HAVE ISSUES"**

1. While addiction is real, many people have gray-area problems with substances that do not fit the criteria for a substance misuse disorder.

2. A good indicator of a substance misuse disorder is that someone who is regularly using substances is not meeting their goals in work or in life.

3. Understanding and working with your nervous system is a great way to prevent developing a substance misuse disorder.

Myth #30: "Therapy Is Not Political"

Believe it or not, therapists are talking about politics with their patients. Many times, clinicians will actually be open about their political beliefs with their patients. One study published in 2019 found that 87 percent of therapists discussed politics with their patients.[1] This means that the vast majority of people talk about politics in therapy. Sixty-three percent of therapists surveyed reported some degree of self-disclosure of their political views. This means that therapists either explicitly explained their political views to their patients or felt that their stances were heavily implied. The researchers found that therapists were more likely to disclose their political views if they perceived their patients were sharing their own political views.

Many therapists justify self-disclosure by pointing to the potential for the therapeutic alliance to get stronger when the therapist reveals something about themselves. That is certainly true in some cases. In other cases, therapists will refrain from self-disclosing to preserve the neutrality of the therapeutic space.

When a patient brings up politics within the context of therapy, however, my first thought is not about self-disclosure. Instead, I tend to suspect that when a patient brings up politics, what's going on with the person may not actually be about politics. This is Psychoanalysis 101: What the patient is thinking about is just the surface-level thought, and the conversation needs to go deeper. In other words, patients may think they need to discuss politics, but they're actually concerned about something else. For example, people come into therapy thinking they need to talk about their dating life, but they often need to talk about their childhood. Or people come into therapy to deal with depression, but the depression actually stems from something else, such as untreated ADHD.

Are the therapists who are encouraging political discussions doing so because it's healing their patients? Or are these discussions healing the therapist?

My suspicion that therapists might have other motivations for disclosing political beliefs comes from the fact that some psychotherapists see themselves more as activists than as practitioners who treat mental illness. Anyone who works in the mental health field knows exactly what I am talking about, because this is not actually a secret. Talkspace is one of the biggest mental health companies, with an estimated worth of about $300 million.[2] The company published an article on its website titled "Therapy Is Political. It's High Time Therapists Acknowledge This."[3] The author, Reina Gattuso, articulates an explanation that is heavily influenced by what I would call a collectivist philosophy.

One way to understand the collectivist perspective is to consider how individuals do not exist in isolation from one another. As one viral video trend put it, when a flower is failing to bloom, do you blame the flower or the quality of the soil, air, or sunshine? The collectivist perspective encourages us to prioritize the patient's community and broader societal structures. Therefore, to a collectivist, it makes sense to advocate for systemic changes through politics. For example, if a patient is experiencing burnout due to economic stress, collectivists would argue that a good response is to advocate for redistributive policies that would give that person relief and alleviate symptoms of burnout. Collectivists argue that unless the systemic barriers and inequalities that impact individuals are tackled, genuine progress with mental health will remain elusive. Collectivists will often be heard talking about politics, systemic change, and social justice when it comes to mental health and other topics due to these broader considerations.

Clinicians who adhere to collectivist tenets believe the project of mental health expands outside the therapy session itself. In the Talkspace article, Gattuso writes, "According to healing justice practitioners, we can only achieve well-being through systemic change." I want to reiterate her word choices of *justice*, *only*, and *systemic change*. Gattuso seems to believe that systemic change is the only way to pursue mental health and justice. You might be tempted to say that one author's article is not indicative of the attitude of an entire field, but Talkspace actually goes as far as to include the following disclaimer: "Articles are extensively reviewed by our team of clinical experts (therapists and psychiatrists of various specialties) to ensure content is accurate and on par with current industry standards." Therefore, I feel justified in asserting that this attitude is widely held among clinicians. It's worth pointing out that Gattuso is not a clinician. She's training to be an anthropologist.[4] Naturally, an anthropologist is going to be biased toward a collectivist approach, because anthropology is the study of culture.

The mental health field is not monolithically collectivist. Many practitioners also prioritize what is called an individualistic approach. Unlike collectivists, individualists champion concepts such as self-determination and free will. They believe that the individual is sacred when it comes to both personal transformation and societal change. They push back on the collectivist outlook by arguing that systems are made up of individuals. The individualists' critique of the flower metaphor is that human beings are not flowers, so the analysis has limited applicability. We can uproot ourselves and change our circumstances. Individualists point out that even if economic reform, as an example of systemic change, could alleviate the symptoms of burnout, that doesn't solve the immediate needs of the person in front of the mental health practitioner. In addition, individualists point out that it is equally unjust to withhold effective treatment from this person while citing systemic advocacy. Individualists believe that the ideas underpinning collectivist philosophy are at complete odds with justice and the ethics of beneficence (how to benefit the patient) and non-maleficence (how to do no harm to the patient).[5] An individualist would say that treating a person like a flower that cannot escape its system is akin to reinforcing codependent and infantilizing dynamics. Such dynamics can keep patients stuck in an unempowered state of consciousness, which some might unnecessarily identify with a victim mentality.

It may not be obvious how the individualistic and collectivist philosophies are necessarily political. If you think about it, the more collectivist you are in your orientation, the more politically you are going to think about your work as a mental health professional. If you truly believe that your ability to provide treatment is greatly limited with the systemic factors at play, why wouldn't you become an activist? To hold collectivist beliefs but not advocate for change would be not only ineffectual but also hypocritical. In its extreme manifestations, some collectivists can be antagonistic to those who do not share their worldview and commitment to action. Many feel that "inaction is just siding with the oppressor," a quote often attributed to bishop and theologian Desmond Tutu. In this case, inaction can be construed as siding with the system and therefore against mental health.

While collectivists make a strong case, it is not one that holds up to scrutiny. The stance that people are either for progress or against progress may be an example of all-or-nothing thinking. In cognitive therapy, all-or-nothing thinking is called cognitive distortion—sometimes referred to as a thinking error.

When it comes to discussing competing philosophies in the mental health field, things can start to feel quite esoteric and abstract. That's why I want to tell you about Amanda, so you can consider these dynamics as they apply to actual patient care. Amanda used to bring up politics a lot during our therapy sessions and would sometimes cry when she thought about economic inequality. In fact, this happened during our sessions several times. She identified as a socialist and believed that a socialist system would solve most of the world's problems. Amanda eventually told me that she had not been honest about everything that was going on with her mental health. She wanted to tell me, but she felt guilty every single time she tried to bring it up to me. When I asked why she felt so guilty, she explained that she was aware that there were so many less privileged people than her. Her problems felt silly compared to their problems, and she felt helpless. Amanda felt she couldn't tell me what was going on with her because so many other people had problems that were so much worse, by her definition. At the same time, Amanda also felt she couldn't do anything, as an individual, to change the systems that, according to her, allowed economic inequality to exist.

I prompted Amanda to consider at what other times in her life she felt guilty for talking about her problems. When else was she encouraged to compare her problems to those of the less fortunate? Her answer was not political in the slightest. Instead, she talked about her parents and her upbringing. She told me that *every single time* she complained about anything growing up, they told her to shut up and be grateful. After all, so many other people had it so much worse than her. What did she have to complain about?

Amanda eventually opened up to me about self-harm behavior. Her emotional pain had been so thoroughly suppressed that she had resorted to cutting herself for an emotional release. Instead of discussing politics or social theory, we were able to do valuable work together. I believe that had I engaged in a political discussion and kept our conversations at an intellectual level, it would have taken Amanda a much longer time to tell me about her self-harm, if she had decided to tell me at all. In the art of psychotherapy, I have learned that timing is almost everything. I believe my timing with Amanda and refraining from self-disclosure helped her to feel comfortable within our nonjudgmental therapeutic space and, eventually, to be open about her mental health concerns.

Over time, as Amanda became more regulated and better able to process her emotions in an adaptive way, she continued to bring up politics. At a certain point, I engaged in self-disclosure about my own political beliefs. I let her know that I didn't share her socialist bona fides. I told Amanda that if I was a socialist, I would feel much better if I felt that my actions were aligned with my values. I told her about how I started my own business—my private practice—due to my beliefs about economics and that it was good for my mental health because I was walking the walk, not just talking the talk. My timing in this self-disclosure felt therapeutically appropriate in that I could model an open conversation in which, though we didn't agree on a specific philosophy, we both were taking steps to enhance our own mental health in ways that aligned with our values. This is something therapists call acceptance and commitment therapy, or ACT. In ACT, you work to increase the alignment between values and behaviors. When people are out of alignment with their values, their mental health usually suffers. When they are engaged in committed action around those values, their mental health improves. Therapists work to help their patients understand how their values impact both their behaviors and their mental health.

Even though we were politically different, I helped Amanda think about things she could do to reform the system according to her beliefs. Eventually, she became very passionate about ethical consumption. She heavily researched how the products she purchased were created and made every effort to purchase from people and companies that aligned with her values. She created lists and spreadsheets, started a blog, and enrolled loved ones in her cause. Amanda also started to volunteer for an environmental nonprofit, another issue that mattered deeply to her. She stopped crying about the state of the world so much. She was better able to focus on what she could control to make the world a better place. The good news was that her mental health improved. Her nervous system was regulated enough so that she could be a better advocate about issues that mattered to her, political and otherwise. I'm very proud of the work Amanda accomplished, both in therapy and outside of it.

Psychobabble

What do you think of Amanda's story? Do you agree with how I handled her case? Would you have done anything differently? A collectivist might argue that I should have engaged Amanda in a discussion about her privilege as it related to systemic change. They might be curious why I did not mention her race or class in my conceptualization of symptoms. A collectivist might point out that I could have engaged her in a conversation about privilege while also utilizing techniques from ACT. Some might even argue that I should have prioritized the conversation about her privilege over the more psychoanalytic lens, which prompted me to learn about her childhood. The authors of the textbook *Counseling the Culturally Diverse*, Drs. Derald Sue and David Sue, would agree.[6] Chapter 2 of the textbook, "The Superordinate Nature of Multicultural Counseling," implies in its title that thinking about a patient like Amanda through a collectivist lens—using a systemic analysis—is superior to trying to help her by considering her childhood the way I did. I respectfully disagree. I viewed Amanda as a whole patient, with equal priority on her lived experiences from childhood to adulthood.

Let me be clear, it's necessary to consider systemic and cultural aspects when understanding anybody or anything, including when developing a treatment plan for psychotherapy. Culture is just one piece of the puzzle. To properly understand mental health problems, you need to conduct a multivariate analysis. A multivariate analysis considers multiple ways to understand the patient's problem, while a univariate analysis considers only one way. Therefore, I think it's incorrect to assert that emphasizing a cultural analysis over a standard multivariate analysis is always the best approach. I actually think the Sues would agree: If you read their textbook, they are emphasizing that when cultural data points are left out, the treatment is incompetent. I wholeheartedly agree.

At the same time, it is inaccurate to assert that I had treated Amanda through a purely individualistic framework. I am neither dogmatically individualistic nor collectivist in my treatment with patients. Furthermore, I would argue that standard psychoanalytic frameworks, such as considering childhood, incorporate a collectivist philosophy by design. Families and childhood are part of the system in which we develop our own unique psychologies. The context through which we exist is more multilayered than the economy and a broad culture. It also includes your subculture, and your family can be considered a subculture. Considering the ethnicity of your family, among other cultural factors, is part of that analysis. Another practitioner could have focused only on alleviating Amanda's symptoms by introducing emotional regulation techniques, ignoring these broader components. Without processing the guilt that stemmed from her childhood context, however, Amanda might have experienced more stress and harm. By discussing her childhood, I was able to synthesize collectivist and individualistic philosophies to provide my patient with the best care I could with the information I had at the time.

Amanda's case has a happy ending, but sometimes I fear that psychotherapists get too attached to their ideologies when it comes to individualistic and collectivist stances. The mental health field is already plagued by so much psychobabble that adding additional philosophical and political dynamics to the mix only confuses things even further. While it's not fun to consider that some therapists may not know where that line is for themselves, it's important that *you* know. In fact, in an informal poll I shared with my followers on Instagram, approximately 30 percent of respondents felt their therapist was too ideologically rigid to give competent therapy. That's not good! I hope the actual number is much smaller, but I am certain the number is not zero. That's why you should know about these dynamics, because your own therapy could be affected by it.

My general stance is to be careful if the therapist is too overly rigid. After all, while systems are made up of individuals, individuals are not separate from the systems in which they exist. If your therapist is unwilling to consider systemic dynamics such as politics, culture, economic factors, and your community, then the therapist might be too ideologically individualistic. If your therapist refuses to think about your problems outside of systemic factors, they might be extremely collectivistic. Such a therapist may even think of themselves more as an activist promoting justice than as a psychotherapist facilitating treatment. I wish I did not have to tell you that. I wish that the therapeutic alliance—the sacred relationship between patient and practitioner—were devoid of the animosity and complexity that is all too often present in these debates. I wish I could tell you these things because most people tend to feel uncomfortable when they learn that their therapist may have politics that differ from their own—and even more unsettled when they learn that their therapist may be allowing their politics or personal philosophies to guide patient care.

Sometimes, I fear my fellow colleagues are more interested in promoting their own collectivist ideology than in helping the person right in front of them. But it's not all bad news that therapists feel so strongly about political and philosophical topics, or that they openly discuss these with patients. The good news is that regardless of how your psychotherapists navigate this debate, most of the time, they are doing it in service of you. They are doing it in service of your mental health care. Each side of the debate is so steadfast in their beliefs because they really care about improving people's lives and helping people improve their mental health and well-being. It's vital to remember that.

Furthermore, your therapist can still favor one side of the debate and be flexible enough to provide competent therapy. Personally, I feel very clear on what my job is as a psychotherapist. I'm here to help people, and in the context of my private practice, I am here to help individuals. That does not make me incapable of considering systemic factors or advocating for systemic change outside of my private practice. Every single person is different, and different cases might require nonidentical treatment approaches. There are plenty of therapists who provide exceptional care, regardless of their politics.

---

3 THINGS TO REMEMBER ABOUT MYTH #30: "THERAPY IS NOT POLITICAL"

1. Therapy can be political because therapists openly discuss politics with patients and may even promote their own ideologies through therapy.

2. The main political debate of the mental health field is between collectivists and individualists.

3. Ideally, patient care combines and integrates aspects of collectivist and individualist frameworks.

Part VI

Shrink Secrets: Common Myths About Therapists

Myth #31: "Therapists Treat Clients, Not Patients"

Some of you might be thinking, *Why does he refer to the people therapists help as patients? Aren't they his clients?* Others might be confused about why a health care professional would refer to the individuals they treat as if the professional were a consultant. While choosing what to call people who seek treatment might seem to be a simple matter of semantics or preference, it highlights a debate that holds profound implications for the mental health field.

Personally, I do not believe that mental health professionals should refer to the people in treatment as clients. Some therapists argue that the word *client* resolves a power imbalance that is implied when the word *patient* is used. They prefer to be collaborative in their therapeutic approach rather than acting from a place of authority. While I certainly see the value in being collaborative with a person you treat only once a week (that person knows themselves better than you do), *there is not a single study that I could find demonstrating that using the term* client *rather than* patient *strengthens the therapeutic alliance, shortens treatment time, or enhances treatment in any meaningful way.* This is a researchable question that seemingly no one has thought to look into.

Second, until society can appreciate mental health to the extent it appreciates physical health, it does not make sense to deemphasize the seriousness of mental illness by calling those who receive treatment for it clients, as if therapists are consultants for a corporation. Many mental health advocates will lament how unfortunate it is that mental health is not treated with the same attention, seriousness, and respect that is given to physical health. Sometimes, these are the same people who advocate against an approach that medicalizes normal human experience. Why do they also insist on framing themselves in a way that takes away from their own importance? Until I can get a cogent response to this concern, and until mental health is respected and funded with the seriousness it deserves, I am going to refer to the people I treat as patients.

Different individuals like to be called patients or clients depending on their own guiding philosophy and personal preferences. I do not believe it meaningfully changes treatment plans for the therapist to defer to the preference of those they are helping, particularly when the preference boils down to semantics. Sometimes, the people I work with in my clinical practice who prefer to be called clients like to refer to their treatment plan as their curriculum. I have no problem with this. You can be called a client and still receive a diagnosis. Some people, when seeking out therapy, feel that the word *patient* might be stigmatizing, because it's a term that denotes someone receiving medical treatment. Starting therapy can be a difficult step to take, and many people fear receiving psychotherapy for the first time because they do not want to feel as though they're "crazy." Others find that the word *client* feels cold and impersonal, as if they are paying for a corporate service rather than receiving some sort of care.

What's my preference? I typically go with what the person sitting in front of me wants, but I default to using the word *patient* because I believe, for now, it helps legitimize the profession.

---

3 THINGS TO REMEMBER ABOUT MYTH #31: "THERAPISTS TREAT CLIENTS, NOT PATIENTS"

1. Different mental health professionals refer to the people they work with as patients or clients for a variety of reasons.

2. There is not a single ounce of research that suggests that either of these terms affects therapy in a meaningful way.

3. If you have a preference, your therapist will likely honor it.

Myth #32: "Therapists Should Never Give Advice"

In the documentary *Stutz*, actor Jonah Hill interviews his therapist about his work as a practitioner.[1] Dr. Phil Stutz comments on the widely held belief that a therapist should never intrude on the patient's process and should never give advice, so the patient can figure things out for themselves. Dr. Stutz finds this perspective "not acceptable." Jonah Hill agrees. In the documentary, he remarks on how helpful therapy has been to him personally: "Your friends who are idiots give you advice. . . . And you want your friends just to listen and you want your therapist to give you advice." Many therapists saw this documentary and were shocked at the heretical nature of these claims. Others, like myself, were ecstatic to see a therapist embrace a more directive and honest approach.

One bad reason for being nondirective that therapists sometimes cite is one of emotional safety. I get where they are coming from, but it's a completely myopic assumption to say that people find nondirective feedback more emotionally safe or comfortable than feedback from someone who is more straight-talking, honest, and in-your-face about what they think. I don't know about you, but in my life, people who are overly polite to the point of being insincere can sometimes make me less comfortable than people who are honest but a tad offensive or inaccurate. There is a cultural consideration here as well. My patients in New York City are accustomed to a certain kind of unapologetic frankness that my patients in Colorado are not always looking for in a therapist.

There are many good reasons, however, that therapists are taught in school to never give advice. I keep these reasons in mind when I am working with patients. The first one is an issue of humility. When you begin therapy, your therapist doesn't know you that well, so they can't give you adequate advice, even if they want to. Many people are frustrated by this dynamic when they start therapy. They complain that the therapist just asks lots of questions or seems to repeat and paraphrase what the patient says to them. Since this is such a common gripe about therapists, I want to tell you what I tell my patients when they start their work with me:

> *The first several sessions I will just be getting to know you, so don't expect any direct feedback, a deep analysis, or much applicable advice. Instead, I will ask lots of questions and repeat back what I think I am hearing to ensure that I know I'm hearing you right. After a while, I will start to be more direct with you, if that's what you want. It might take some time, but the quality of therapy will be much improved if you allow me a little patience as we get our start.*

I didn't always proceed this way with patients. When I began practicing as a therapist, like many young practitioners, I was so eager to give feedback that I would sometimes "rush to restore." What an inexperienced therapist often will do is rush in with advice or an analysis; this feedback is usually not helpful, because they do not know the patient well enough yet. Their advice is based on too many assumptions and is ultimately not applicable.

Another good reason that therapists are told never to give advice is that sometimes the advice patients need the most is the hardest for them to accept. It's easier for them to swallow that advice if they come to the conclusion on their own. Best case, the advice may fall on deaf ears. Worst case, it can actually run the risk of making the patient less open to feedback if the advice is given before they are ready to hear it.

When Sara came to see me, she reported feeling depressed and unmotivated. She also disclosed that she was smoking marijuana every single day. I immediately advised her to stop smoking weed for a short period, to see whether it was connected to her depressive symptoms. Sara really did not want to stop. I did not know for sure that her cannabis misuse was connected to her depressive symptoms, but it was important to rule that possibility out. I could be the best therapist in the world and the best fit for Sara, but if she was feeling depressed because she smoked weed every morning and every night, no amount or quality of therapy was going to help.

Many people would agree that it's practical to rule out the role that cannabis might play in someone's depressive symptoms before trying cognitive behavioral therapy. In this case, I saw little risk in being direct with Sara. The worst thing that could happen did happen, and it wasn't that bad. She simply let me know she was not interested in stopping consuming cannabis in the morning. Over time, as she got frustrated by her lack of progress in therapy, she slowly became more open to the idea that smoking weed in the morning was affecting her energy levels and motivation.

That's the thing about advice. Sometimes, it's obvious, and it needs to be said. For example, when I treated Jimmy, he was experiencing all sorts of mental dysfunction. He couldn't think clearly. He couldn't finish sentences. In my first session with him, I found out he was malnourished. Jimmy didn't have an eating disorder; he just needed to be reminded that everyone needs more than a few hundred calories a day. That's the thing about depression. It can cause you to forget to eat and drink enough water and bathe with an appropriate frequency. But neglecting to eat, drink, or bathe can also make you feel depressed. In Jimmy's case, when he started eating more, his depression symptoms didn't go away, but they immediately improved. It made the rest of therapy easier knowing that his body was being adequately nourished. Personally, I think it would be unethical to say that I shouldn't or couldn't give him that advice or that it would be therapeutically risky to give that advice.

There is a huge difference between giving advice and being direct or being honest. Sometimes, what I think patients mean when they say they wish their therapist would give them better advice is that they feel their therapist is not being direct or honest with them. It's been my experience that honesty is curative. Even if the feedback is something that the patient is "not ready to hear," I find that if our rapport is good, they will tell me they disagree. I like it when my patients disagree with me. It's often the case that I am missing an important piece of context. Sometimes, I assess that my patient simply isn't ready to accept something emotionally difficult. That's still good data for me to know, so I find that being direct can usually be fruitful.

Rather than describing myself as a therapist who gives lots of advice—though I am certainly not afraid to do so—it might be more accurate to say that I'm a therapist who is not afraid to be honest or direct with the people in his care. Don't fool yourself; honesty in therapy can be scary. For example, I don't ever give advice on whether my patient should continue to date the person they are seeing, but I will, if clinically appropriate, be honest with them about what comes up for me when they complain about how their partner treats them. For example, if I am hearing stories about how my patient is being physically abused or treated unfairly, I may share how that makes me feel. It doesn't matter whether the patient is biased in their telling of the story—what matters is that it may be clinically effective to be that direct with them. That sort of honesty can be difficult but is usually productive and even curative.

---

3 THINGS TO REMEMBER ABOUT MYTH #32: "THERAPISTS SHOULD NEVER GIVE ADVICE"

1. There are times when giving advice is perfectly therapeutically appropriate.

2. There is a difference between a therapist giving you advice and a therapist being more honest and transparent about their thoughts on your situation.

3. Honesty can be productive and curative.

Myth #33: "Therapists Psychoanalyze Everyone They Meet"

In a previous relationship, I distinctly remember going on a double date with my boyfriend's friends. Over dinner, one of them joked about how, being a therapist, I must be psychoanalyzing my partner all the time. I was offended but tried to play it off with humor. My boyfriend just laughed, but I remember his friend as a very straightforward and honest person. With zero judgment, she simply locked eyes with me and said, "It's not like you can help it. It's what you do for a living." Is she right? Are therapists constantly analyzing the people around them?

The number one question I get as a therapist is "Do you psychoanalyze the people you date?" In the first phase of my career, this question brought me a good amount of personal anxiety. I used to reply, "Don't worry, you never do something you're good at for free," or "Don't worry, you're too well-adjusted for me to be interested in what's happening in your head." People usually laugh at these deflections, so I sometimes still use them. When I was in grad school, I remember often feeling vigilant about this dynamic. It came up not just in dating, but with all my loved ones and everyone I would meet. I remember feeling it was really important to me that not only did I not *sound* like a therapist when I talked to others, but I did not even *think* like one in social situations. Thinking like a therapist was work, and I didn't want to work in my personal life.

They say hindsight is 20/20 vision. In hindsight, I actually wish I had felt more permission to think like a therapist in my personal life. I wish I had allowed myself to trust my gut and my hard-earned clinical intuition when picking a partner or deciding whether a new acquaintance was worthy of becoming a true friend. My issue was not so much that I constantly analyzed the people in my life; my issue was that I was disconnecting with a part of myself—the part who is a practicing psychotherapist—and making judgments and decisions about people without the help of that part of myself. I would overlook obvious red flags because I was ignoring my inner practitioner, who could see the warning signs. I did so to avoid the stigma associated with being a mental health professional.

Of course, I don't want to imply that therapists never make mistakes or cannot be erroneous in their assessments of their patients or loved ones. Of course they can. I must admit, though, as I have gotten older and more seasoned as a therapist and person, my judgments have sharpened as I give myself permission to think like a therapist whenever it's helpful to do so. The truth is that everyone analyzes the people they date. The vast majority of people observe the behavior of people in their lives and conduct themselves based on how they interpret that data.

These days, whenever people ask me if I analyze everyone I date, I have a different answer for them. "Of course I do. Don't you?" This answer usually gets a laugh, because it's true. In fact, if you're not assessing your date, you're probably not doing it correctly. Everyone is analyzing one another all the time. In business, everyone is constantly attempting to know one another's intentions and levels of trustworthiness. In dating, people often enlist the help of trusted friends to analyze the meaning of ambiguous texts or interpret strange behavior. In intimacy, there is a desire to deeply know your loved ones, to be seen, and this process often is assisted by disclosing childhood wounds and past experiences. Whether you want to admit it or not, therapists are not the only ones analyzing the people in their lives. We're just the only ones who get called out on it.

One of the more subtle ways psychobabble confuses people about the correct and incorrect use of psychological jargon was just displayed in this chapter. I used the verb *to psychoanalyze* to mean "to psychologically interpret" someone. That is how the word is used by most people, including some therapists. The truth is, you cannot properly conduct psychoanalysis in your personal relationships. The craft of psychoanalysis, in both its classical and modern-day manifestations, requires an objective party. While all therapists are people, and all people have biases, removing the personal relationship piece allows for greater objectivity because the personal biases and motives are lessened. When I say that "everybody analyzes everybody," what I mean is that everyone is observing one another's behavior and speech and inferring conclusions based on those observations.

Furthermore, therapy is not as analytical as some people think. It is not often a profound analysis that heals my patients. It is often the simple reflections that trigger a touch of self-awareness and ultimately catalyze the healing process. Being told by your therapist that you're spoiled, that you're resentful, that you were neglected, or that something about your childhood you thought was normal wasn't normal at all—these are things that often have a profound impact on my patients. The same is true in personal life. The times I have offered my analysis of loved ones, I have often been told to "stop talking like a shrink." But when I have been authentic and compassionate, and simply reflected what I was seeing and feeling, I have had the most powerful interactions with my loved ones. As in therapy, as in life—doing your best to be a good human seems to be the crux of the work.

I am not perfect at navigating professional boundaries in my personal life. I don't think most people are. The truth is, my shrink brain is not something I turn on or off like a light switch. It's not a dial that I turn up and down between 0 and 100 percent depending on the person I'm talking to. It's a part of me, just as what you do is part of you. I have a dear friend who is a teacher, and sometimes he offers comments in an instructive tone that I don't always appreciate. My friends in finance refer to our relationship implicitly in terms of costs and benefits. I have a friend who is in law enforcement, and I always feel like they're interrogating me. The truth is, the jobs we have can and do affect the ways our minds work. Furthermore, when I interpret a friend's behavior, they don't immediately associate it with my job, because they can't. I give my friends grace, regardless of their profession, and hope they give it back to me in return.

The funny thing is that psychotherapists often deal with the stigma of supposedly analyzing everyone all the time or wanting to hear about a stranger's problems. Yet, among therapists, the joke we often tell each other is to never be honest about what you do for a living to someone you're sitting next to on a plane. All too often, when we tell the wrong person what we do, they are more than happy to disclose their mental health history. The last place you want to be is on a flight seated next to a person who is looking for free advice or a sympathetic ear. When I meet a dating prospect, I typically hear jokes about how they want me to fix them just as often as I hear jokes about how I better not analyze them. Personally, both responses make me curious about whether those jokes are coming from a deeper place. But I don't want to overthink things.

I think I can speak on behalf of mental health professionals everywhere when I say that whether you want us to ignore the obvious signs of your undiagnosed condition or want to hear our opinion, the truth is we're not going to give you our thoughts if you don't ask for them. And even then, we likely won't give them to you, because you're not our patient. At the same time, I think most therapists would agree with me and say that it's always disappointing when a loved one mentions they haven't been honest with me about their struggles because they don't want to overburden me. While I appreciate the consideration, I am often a little offended that the implication is that I don't care about the relationship enough to view it outside of the scope of work. If you're my loved one and you're reading this, of course I am here for you. I will be honest if work was too draining for me to be as supportive as I would like to be with you.

> **3 THINGS TO REMEMBER ABOUT MYTH #33:
> "THERAPISTS PSYCHOANALYZE
> EVERYONE THEY MEET"**
>
> **1.** Everyone analyzes one another to a certain degree.
>
> **2.** Proper psychoanalysis cannot take place outside the therapy room.
>
> **3.** Being a therapist does not require engaging in deep analysis—just being honest and reflective.

Myth #34: "Shrinks Are Crazier than Their Patients"

When I was in graduate school, at the beginning of every semester, each student would introduce themselves and engage in some sort of icebreaker activity. Invariably, people would be asked why they wanted to become a therapist. When I first started school, I always carried a private judgment about one particular answer. Many times, one of my fellow classmates would answer that question with some version of the following: "I want to be a therapist because I want to treat survivors of intense physical and emotional abuse."

I remember wondering what kind of person would aspire to do that for their job every day and whether these people might even have needed a little bit of therapy themselves. What else could explain their affinity to listening to such heartbreaking stories all day? Then I began to learn about trauma, abuse, family systems, and psychodynamic theory, and before long, I too became very invested in those kinds of cases. I sometimes compare this to the situation of a surgeon working in the emergency room. Sure, surgeons are faced with treating horrific injuries, but they receive satisfaction when they save lives. If that's your craft, it's normal to want a challenge. Many therapists have treated standard anxiety and depression. As our skills develop, many of us are interested in more challenging cases.

The stigma that is associated with working in the mental health field is understandable. Most people imagine the work as intellectually exhausting, energetically overstimulating, and emotionally draining. People imagine what it must be like to facilitate therapy all day long and assume that for someone to enjoy that work means there must be something wrong with them. Another popular assumption is that people go into mental health because they unconsciously want to fix themselves. There is also the wounded healer archetype, which is about a person who has chosen to become a therapist due to their history of mental illness or surviving some sort of significant struggle in their lives.

It's true that some clinicians would be better suited to receive much more therapy than they provide, but there is no substantial evidence to support the stereotype that statistically more therapists have mental health concerns than the rest of the population. I have to confess that I do wonder, since psychologists are designing these studies, whether there is an inherent bias making me and my colleagues look better than we deserve to. At the same time, evidence *does* show that there are higher rates of psychopathy and narcissism in media, sales, law, surgery, and politics. If you believe that shrinks are crazier than their patients, but you feel fine with hanging out with people in those professions, you would be wise to consider not *whether* they're crazy but *how* they're crazy. Is it a flavor of crazy that you want to have in your life?

In my line of work, *crazy* is a meaningless word. For one thing, the definition of *crazy* has expanded to encapsulate both atypical *and* normative behavior. There are more than 150 different mental health diagnoses in the Diagnostic and Statistical Manual of Mental Disorders. That doesn't even include all the subclinical, nondiagnostic distinctions used to describe psychological phenomena. For example, impostor syndrome is not mentioned once in the DSM-V, but it's still a common experience and something that can improve with therapy or some other type of support. Lots of times, what we call mental disorders are normative reactions to stressful circumstances. For example, developing social anxiety after a series of social rejections does not make you crazy—it makes you a person.

The promise of the mental health field is not about delineating what constitutes psychopathology or clinically significant dysfunction. The promise of the mental health field is about unlocking one's sense of agency and freedom. When you are depressed and the phone rings, depression will say something like "What's the point of getting up to answer the phone right now?" When you are anxious, and everything is going well, anxiety will say something like "The thing you forgot to worry about is definitely going to happen now because you can't remember it." Through treatment, you can be liberated from these constraints, so you can answer the phone and you can be more present without excessive worrying.

Those who work in the mental health field are not unlike doctors who need someone to do their surgery or hairdressers who need someone else to trim their neckline. I see nothing wrong with people who work in mental health needing that external support. In fact, many practitioners believe that it's easier to empathize and connect with patients if you've been in the vulnerable position of requiring therapy yourself.

Are shrinks crazy? They can be. Are they crazier than their patients? Definitely sometimes. For me, the far more interesting question is how they got into this work. I can only speak for myself. I believe the answer is partly biological or even spiritual. I could make stuff up about being gay, my dad dying, receiving a ton of therapy after his death, or having a temperament that makes me well suited for the work. I could tell you that I'm innately curious, compassionate, and analytical. I could explain that I am a very verbal person, so I like having a job that lets me talk to people all day. If you asked my mom, she'd tell you that when I was very young, if she and my dad were arguing, I would watch them. I would get Post-it notes, tally the behaviors that I observed, and give them their reports. I honestly don't even believe that story when she tells it; it's too incredible. When I let her know I wanted to go to grad school, that was the story she told me in response. I don't think you can attribute that tendency of mine to trauma or upbringing in any serious way. It's something deeper.

I want to leave you with an alternative hypothesis about why people go into the mental health profession. It has been my observation that many of my colleagues grew up with a family member or loved one who struggled with mental health issues. Perhaps it was a sibling, perhaps it was a girlfriend or boyfriend in high school. Perhaps it was a good family friend. Whatever the case may be, many therapists I have gotten to know have described an experience of learning, from a young age, how to have compassion with someone who is struggling. Think about it: For children who have grown up with a parent who has a mood disorder, it makes sense that a way to cope might be to develop deep empathy and understanding for that parent. If you grew up giving a loved one that kind of grace and patience and love, it would make transitioning to the work of a therapist very easy.

Are therapists crazier than their patients? It depends on how you define crazy. That's not a cop-out. If mental health culture can agree on one thing, among all the psychobabble that plagues it, it's that *crazy* is an unspecific, unhelpful, and meaningless word.

---

3 THINGS TO REMEMBER ABOUT MYTH #34: "SHRINKS ARE CRAZIER THAN THEIR PATIENTS"

1. Some therapists are crazier than their patients, while some are not.

2. *Crazy* is a meaningless word; try to be more specific when you're claiming someone is crazy.

3. Some therapists become interested in the field because a loved one struggled with mental illness, not necessarily because they themselves have a mental health condition.

Myth #35: "Therapists Never Talk About Themselves with Patients"

"What are your politics?!" That was the question my patient, Brenna, yelled at me as she sat down to begin our session. She was so angry and exasperated. Truthfully, I was surprised. Brenna exhibited a gentle demeanor and came across as fairly unopinionated about most topics. She was a ski bum in the winter months and a summer camp counselor in the summer months. She had a happy-go-lucky attitude and was generally uninterested in talking about dark or intense subjects. She initially sought out therapy for PTSD following an accident on a mountain bike. The question about politics seemed to come out of nowhere.

Like any good therapist, I didn't rush into self-disclosure about my political beliefs. *Self-disclosure* is the term therapists use to mean telling patients about themselves. Instead, I got curious. I asked her, "Why does this feel so urgent today?" It was June 2022, and she had just heard that *Roe v. Wade* had been overturned by the US Supreme Court. *Roe v. Wade* was the ruling that guaranteed abortion access at the federal level in the United States. Brenna explained that she didn't actually want to hear about my politics. She just couldn't bear the thought of me "celebrating," in my personal life, this judicial ruling. I learned that she had strong feelings about being pro-choice, partly informed by her decision to get an abortion when she was a teenager. I let her know that I did not celebrate the ruling. I asked Brenna whether she felt she needed to know more about my beliefs on abortion. Arguably, one could be pro-life and still not celebrate the ruling with the sort of glee she was imagining. I wanted to make sure she wasn't seeking something else out of the conversation. Brenna let me know she was satisfied with the fact that I wasn't celebratory. She reported feeling better, and we proceeded with her course of treatment for her PTSD.

Have you ever asked your therapist about their political beliefs? You're allowed to ask your therapist about anything you want, including their politics. Your therapist has the right to not answer you, and they may have good reasons for disclosing or not disclosing different aspects of themselves. If you are fiercely pro-choice, like Brenna, would you have rushed in to let her know you agree on the topic? Would that have been a good intervention? Would that have strengthened your therapeutic alliance? If you are pro-life, how would you have handled her question? More important, would you have noticed that this dynamic was likely born out of a desire to feel secure in the therapeutic relationship?

Self-disclosure is tricky, whether it's about politics or something else. One variable that should be considered is timing. If a patient you've been treating for five years asks you something personal about yourself, is it the same dynamic as if a patient asked you the same question in their first session? For example, in consults for couples therapy, patients have asked me whether I am married or have ever been married. What would you say? I have colleagues who primarily treat couples. Some of them talk about their marriage on their website. These clinicians self-disclose in their marketing as a way to be relatable to their target market clientele. I have other colleagues who take off their wedding rings before sitting down with their patients, regardless of whether they are seeing a couple or an individual. If you are single and a couples therapist, and the therapy is going well, does your answer to the question about whether you're married or not help things or just unnecessarily introduce a messy dynamic?

When I was in school, I was afraid to self-disclose to my patients. In fact, I almost never told my patients anything about myself. If they asked me something, I would respond in the classic therapist way: "Why is it important for you to know that?" Personally, I felt discouraged from self-disclosing in my training. This makes sense to me because the art of therapeutic conversation is solely about the patient; it is a very one-sided dynamic, for good reason. As I got older and more seasoned in the practice of therapy, I noticed that my supervisors and peer consultations encouraged self-disclosure, in contrast to my graduate training. I have two theories about why.

First, less experienced therapists do not have the self-awareness or clinical dexterity to navigate self-disclosure with skillfulness. Over time, they are able to be less rigid and can self-disclose when doing so might benefit the patient in some way. Second, being a blank slate and never showing any emotion or revealing anything about yourself is one way of doing therapy. Many consider this to be the old-school way of conducting psychoanalysis. More recent contributors to the craft of psychotherapy have noted that it can greatly benefit the patient to see authentic expressions of emotion and to learn about their therapist in strategic ways. For example, in addiction treatment, it can often be really empowering to learn that your therapist also struggled with substance misuse and is successfully in recovery. That information can enhance feelings of closeness and decrease levels of shame in the person who is just struggling to admit they have a problem.

How does your therapist think about self-disclosing or not disclosing? Self-disclosures should always benefit the patient and not the practitioner. To simplify, if the self-disclosure benefits the patient, you can consider revealing personal details to a patient. If there is a risk of harm or if the self-reveal is more about the therapist's own "stuff," then it should be avoided. Of course that's much easier to understand in theory than it is to carry out in practice. Some researchers have studied self-disclosure, but in my opinion, this is an area where psychotherapy becomes as much craft as science, like the practice of medicine or law.

As I have gotten older, I find that I self-disclose frequently but always intentionally. It's always in the back of my mind that I could misread the situation. For example, some people love for their therapist to mention things about themselves. Many patients love it when I share my opinion or let them know I also have struggled in dating or in life. Lots of people feel that self-disclosure by the therapist helps the patient feel they are just talking to another person, which in turn helps them feel close and let their guard down. It enhances a sense of safety. Other times, people respond to hearing about their therapist's opinions or experiences as a violation. All of a sudden, the session has become about the therapist. Some experience this sudden shift in the dynamic as the opposite of emotional safety.

Regardless of your preference, it's always helpful to communicate it to your therapist if they are not intuitively assessing the style you prefer. You are also allowed to change your mind and have your preference vary based on context. For example, if you are processing a traumatic event, that may not be the right time to hear that your therapist has survived something similar. If you are grieving the loss of a loved one, perhaps it would be comforting to hear that your practitioner has experienced similar pain. On the flip side, maybe the person who's grieving doesn't want to hear about anyone else. Maybe they need a therapeutic alliance in which they can be totally and unapologetically focused on themselves and their emotions. Everyone is different.

---

3 THINGS TO REMEMBER ABOUT MYTH #35: "THERAPISTS NEVER TALK ABOUT THEMSELVES WITH PATIENTS"

1. When therapists talk about themselves with patients, sometimes it's great for the therapy process; other times, it hinders the therapeutic process.

2. You are always allowed to communicate to your therapist about your preferences concerning self-disclosure.

3. You are allowed to ask your therapist anything about themselves, but they may have good reasons for not answering your questions.

Part VII

Relational Ruckus: Common Myths That Hurt Your Relationships

Myth #36: "Your Date Is Love-Bombing You"

Do you remember the first time you fell in love with someone? Do you recall the first time you had a crush? The first time you were overcome by lust and desire? Maybe you saw the other person from a certain angle, in the perfect lighting? Perhaps it was something about their sound, their scent or feel, or the prospect of their smell or touch that completely overpowered you? We all can feel out of control when it comes to our experiences with love and desire. The desire does not even need to be sexual in nature. It can be about wanting to feel close to the other person. It can be about the desire to be in love.

We all want and deserve love, so it's no wonder that some people use this basic human need as a way to manipulate others. "Love-bombing" is a psychologically abusive tactic that involves showering someone with excessive affection with the intention to gain control over the other person. It almost always occurs at the early stages of the relationship. The general idea is that if the person is tricked, they will become emotionally invested and attached. Anyone who has been in love knows that it's difficult to see things objectively when you're emotionally attached to someone. Some love-bombers attempt to rush intimacy so they can discover personal details about you in order to be more knowledgeable and better manipulate you in the future. Once this happens, the control and abuse can begin to take shape because you are emotionally invested and they know a lot about you.

Love-bombing is a real tactic. It's important to know what it is, but as a psychotherapist, I have treated both survivors of love-bombing and people who simply move too fast in relationships. Love-bombing and moving too fast are not the same things. It's really important to be clear on the underlying motivation for someone who is moving too quickly. It can be tempting to write off anyone who moves too fast as abusive or unstable, but that judgment isn't always accurate. I also want to be clear and say I am not condoning or justifying moving at lightning speed, but I am encouraging you to be curious about why some people do move that fast. Love-bombing is just one possibility out of many. For example, was Ted Mosby love-bombing Robin Scherbatsky in *How I Met Your Mother*? Ted was an imperfect person as a protagonist. He was flawed and made many mistakes in his love life, but that hardly makes him an abusive love-bomber. Anyone who has seen the television series knows that he did fall fast and hard for her, and he even, technically, ends up with her in the end.

The number one reason why people move too fast is not because they are love-bombing you. Most of the time people move quickly because they want to indulge the fantasy of being in love. Think about it: People often say that falling in love is one of the best things that can happen to you. "Life's greatest prize" is what they call it. It's understandable that some people want to manufacture that feeling, particularly if they are lonely and haven't met someone they liked in a long time. The psychoanalytical interpretation of what happens when you fall for someone is that you *project* an ideal onto them. Typically, your idealized romantic partner is informed by your past experiences—your family, friends, and past relationships. Put another way, the projection consists of assumptions you make to fill in the gaps—knowledge you don't yet have about the other person. When you fall fast, you have essentially fallen for a fantasy. It's a fantasy because you do not know the person all that well yet.

    Falling for someone quickly, projecting an ideal onto them, does not make you damaged or weak or mentally ill. It happens to everyone. In fact, I would go as far as to say that I am not sure people would find love at all if it weren't for this little psychological quirk. It's arguably a good thing to be incentivized to push forward for the sake of love, even though it may not be totally logical. The issue is that sometimes people don't have the life experience to be measured and sober in how they conduct themselves in light of these feelings. Sometimes, feelings can be intense. Sometimes, people's expectations get too high, and they set themselves up to fail. What can happen when people dive headfirst into a relationship is that they end up feeling quite disoriented after a while, when their lover inevitably does not live up to the ideal projected onto them. A breakup can swiftly follow that can leave one or both parties feeling hurt. Just because the initial attraction was informed by a fantasy—a projection—that doesn't mean the feelings for the other person were not real. That kind of pattern certainly doesn't constitute the premeditated manipulation that occurs in love-bombing.

Another reason for moving quickly in a new relationship is the result of neurodivergency. People with ADHD can struggle with hyperfocus. They can have an intense concentration on their new crush that goes above and beyond how a neurotypical brain might think about their new crush often. Hyperfocusing on a new crush, combined with a neurodevelopmental condition that increases levels of impulsivity, can easily lead to behaviors similar to love-bombing. Someone with ADHD may blurt out words of affection, like "I love you." They may buy gifts or demonstrate their interest in other ways, without pausing to think about whether it's too early. That's what impulsivity is—acting without thinking. Some practitioners who work with those on the autism spectrum have told me they have noticed their patients also have a tendency to hyperfocus on a new love interest, but it may be better explained as a hyperfixation. People on the autism spectrum are known to become fixated on various topics or activities. It doesn't seem like a stretch to consider that they might do the same thing with people they are interested in romantically.

There are so many reasons people rush love that are not connected to love-bombing. Colloquially referred to as experiencing "puppy love," people who are younger are often known to dive headfirst into a relationship. Are we really going to label the twelve-year-old who recently entered puberty and got stung by Cupid's arrow for the first time a love-bomber? They're children; it's cute. Let them be. Here's another reason: Have we become so jaded in the age of dating apps that we can't be-

Psychobabble

lieve that sometimes people fall fast and hard and it's genuine? People have reported experiencing this throughout history, and I don't think it's fair to say that they're love-bombing in an intentional way.

In my research for this chapter, I was delighted to find one poll about love-bombing. Shane Co. found that 70 percent of respondents have had their romantic interest say "I love you" within one month of dating.[1] Personally, I do think that's fast. Interestingly, they also found that 66 percent of respondents would rather date a love-bomber than someone who won't or can't commit because they are emotionally unavailable. I am not sure of the poll's methodology because it was not available. It does highlight an interesting question: Are the people who were interviewed so keen on finding love that they would rather be with an abuser than someone who is noncommittal? Or is the entire poll invalid because the respondents do not differentiate love-bombing from moving too quickly? That's the issue with all this psychobabble. If we are not clear on terms and what they mean, the research and data we get when we try to learn about different phenomena will be useless.

There's another common and profound reason for rushing intimacy that may surprise you: Often, people rush intimacy to avoid intimacy. That sounds a little confusing, so let's walk through it.

Sometimes, for whatever reason, people are afraid of feeling close, of feeling true intimacy with someone they are dating. Intimacy can be scary because the person will come to know everything about you, including the things you don't even like to admit to yourself about yourself. One way to avoid that is to rush intimacy and manufacture a feeling of closeness and then stay there. It's a little like rushing into the shallow end of the pool and never going into the deep end. People who rush intimacy in this way can successfully stay in the shallow end of the pool. They can enjoy the intimacy they manufactured through rushing. Inevitably, though, as you get to know a person better over time, you will drift toward the deeper end of the pool. The intimacy will eventually get deeper, more intense, more real, but because the person rushed it, they set themselves up for failure. The advantage to going at a slower pace is you can build a foundation of familiarity and trust, so when the intimacy gets challenging, you have that foundation to fall back on. Usually, though not always, people who rush intimacy to avoid intimacy will exit the relationship if the foundation is too unstable. Closeness built on a fantasy is not true intimacy.

I want to be careful to clarify that slower does not always mean better when it comes to finding love or building sustainable intimacy. While some people do well to go slow, other people meet their partner, get married shortly afterward, and stay together for the rest of their lives. Everyone's experience is different. There is no road map for the journey of love.

The appeal of using love-bombing as a red or yellow flag in dating, to help you sift through the different potential partners in your life, is that it may provide a sense of control. But it's not the most helpful tool. The main way it's helpful is to remind you to have your eyes wide open when things are moving fast. As I have covered in this chapter, the other person may or may not be love-bombing you. Whatever their motivation might be, it's good to develop a deeper and accurate understanding so you can make the most informed decision about what to do next.

3 THINGS TO REMEMBER ABOUT MYTH #36: "YOUR DATE IS LOVE-BOMBING YOU"

1. Love-bombing is an intentional, psychologically abusive act.

2. For someone to rush intimacy does not necessarily mean they are love-bombing you.

3. There are alternative explanations for rushing intimacy. Often, but not always, the behavior isn't fully intentional.

Myth #37: "Freak in the Head, Freak in the Bed"

Every adolescent boy has heard the joke told in a locker room: "Freak in the head, freak in the bed" means that if she's *crazy*, the sex is better. At least, it's the kind of sexual experience you would want to try once. The implication, of course, is that if a person is mentally healthy then the sex must be boring or bland. Interestingly, I have found that there is a parallel stereotype for men, although I am not sure whether it is as widely circulated. Two viral memes echo the same sentiment for the idea that men with mental illness have greater sex appeal. "Depressed boys give the best dick" and "You have mental illness? The D must be fire" have been widely shared on different social media platforms. Everyone knows the trope of how girls pick the bad boy with problems over the nice guy. What does all this mean? Put another way: Is mental illness sexy? If these jokes are funny, and I am not saying that they are, do they have any truth to them?

I don't believe that this myth holds up to scrutiny, but I want to explain why people may believe it to be true. First, I think about bipolar spectrum disorders. In mania or hypomania, people experience an abundance of energy. One of the symptoms is hypersexuality. In a manic or hypomanic phase, people experiencing hypersexuality display an unusually excessive interest in sexual activity. They may take greater risks in choices about the people they have sex with or the types of sexual activity that they engage in. I could see how, to the person they are having sex with, the abundance of energy present in mania or hypomania could seem particularly exciting. The issue is that mania and hypomania can feel fun in the moment but almost always lead to devastating consequences. My clinical opinion is that the trade-off is not worth it. Furthermore, people can become psychotic and delusional in mania. I would be concerned about issues of consent when it comes to sexually engaging with someone who is in a manic state.

    I also think about psychopathy. Someone who is psychopathic does not necessarily have a sense of self in the same way a non-psychopathic person has a sense of self. Someone who is psychopathic thrives on successfully manipulating others. They do not feel emotions the same way other people do. I could imagine that sex with a psychopath would be quite enjoyable if their intention was to fulfill your fantasies so they could manipulate you in some way. If they give you the exact experience you want in bed, you might overlook the obvious warning signs of their psychopathy.

    I recall a patient who briefly dated someone my patient believed had antisocial personality disorder. I was struck by how my patient described the sex: Their erotic interests were perfectly matched. It's not just that they had a lot of overlap in terms of sexual compatibility; it was that everything she wanted and liked was everything he wanted and enjoyed. Does that sound fishy to you? In hindsight, my patient was able to see how especially intense sexual experiences were often paired with other sadistic games they would play. Was the sex especially good? Yes. Was it worth it, given that it was just a sadistic game to the other person? No. There are other ways to get your fantasies fulfilled that do not include engaging with someone with psychopathic features.

Many mental illnesses are not like mania or psychopathy. In depression, one of the main symptoms is called anhedonia, which means you have a hard time experiencing joy and pleasure. Some people even display an outright lack of interest in things that previously brought them joy and pleasure. Sexuality is a site of pleasure and joy for many people, so the idea that depressed people are somehow good in bed does not make much sense. The same thing goes for anxiety. An intense preoccupation that something terrible might happen in the future does not make good sex impossible, but I have a hard time seeing how it raises the chances of the sex being better than usual. It did occur to me that people who are using sex to self-medicate or manage symptoms of a mental illness might seem appealing because they would be particularly eager to engage in the act of sex if they were primarily using it for emotional regulation. That presupposes that desperation and eagerness always lead to being better in bed. While that might be true for some, I am not sure that's true for everyone. Furthermore, *only* using sex as a means for emotional regulation is a risk factor in developing a sex addiction, sometimes called out-of-control sexual behavior. There are many reasons to pursue sex that have nothing to do with managing unpleasant feelings.

I have also wondered if this myth comes not from a belief that a diagnosable condition makes one skillful in the bedroom, but from a belief that people with relational wounds approach sex differently. If someone has a troubled relationship with their family, it's understandable if they approach finding a partner with an elevated level of importance and intention. Most people want to connect with others and experience physical intimacy, but I am talking about something that goes above and beyond what most people do. The stereotype that people discuss is that a woman with "daddy issues" may be extra eager to please someone in bed because it's her way of getting approval and a stable relationship from a man. First of all, however, not everyone is the same when it comes to their erotic selves. Not everyone with childhood baggage approaches sex in this way. Some people's parental baggage actually manifests in the opposite way, and they are fearful of sex. Furthermore, people enjoy giving pleasure just as much as receiving it, if not more so. The idea that someone is extra eager to please may not be appealing to some.

One could argue that someone who is "a freak" is more desirable in bed because a person who struggles with mental illness or emotional problems could be easier to manipulate. I know that might sound unusual and cruel, so I want to explain why that may be possible in at least some situations. In her book *Sexy but Psycho: How the Patriarchy Uses Women's Trauma Against Them*, Dr. Jessica Taylor lays out an argument based on the premise that our society objectifies women as sex objects.[1] Why are women with mental illness sexy? Dr. Taylor argues that women with a mental illness "might be 'psycho' enough to do whatever a man wants them to do." If she's hot and crazy, that's great, but if she's crazy and unattractive, then what value does she offer men? And if she's too crazy, you can hook up with her, but do not marry her; simply manipulate her so you can enjoy yourself and marry someone else. Do you feel gross reading that? I feel gross writing it. And yet this is a thought process for some people, so I feel I have to write about it. It's important to consider when addressing this myth about mental instability and sex appeal.

When those who propagate the myth "freak in the head, freak in the bed" do so out of a desire to manipulate women, the myth certainly holds harmful implications for women, to say the least. I also think there are harmful implications for men, particularly regarding their sex lives. While having a woman act as an "object" to fulfill carnal desires may hold a certain appeal, it's not the only way to be sexually satisfied. In fact, I would argue that's an immature outlook on how to maximize pleasure during sexual activity. Learning to connect, exploring fantasies, and even experiencing yourself as the "object" can be intensely pleasurable. Objectification is not necessarily a bad thing, provided it's consensual. Furthermore, we can apply a feminist framework to look at ways men with mental illness or emotional instability might be more sexually appealing. I wonder whether Dr. Taylor would agree with me that women are often treated as caregivers and that dynamic can contribute to them going after men they can "mother," "fix," "take care of," or "help." There is likely some truth to that for many people. I have a hard time seeing how, if someone's mental health problems are tied to their mother, that makes them more likely to rock your world. Whether you're talking about men or women, we would all be wise to consider how to avoid propagating harmful stereotypes as we discuss these topics.

We don't need to have a purely feminist motivation to want to retire the myth that mental illness is sexy. It's preferable, I believe, to circulate the story that therapy and mental health will improve your sex life. Instead of using psychobabble to convince people that mental illness is sexy, maybe we should instead talk about how mental health is sexy. We should talk about how being aware of your feelings, being authentic in what turns you on, and being able to navigate psychological complexity signal high levels of erotic intelligence.

And if we are going to continue saying that mental illness is sexy, let's do it with the intention of destigmatizing people with mental illness. Even though someone struggles, they can still rock your world in a sane, sexy, and consensual way.

> **3 THINGS TO REMEMBER ABOUT MYTH #37: "FREAK IN THE HEAD, FREAK IN THE BED"**
>
> 1. Mental illness is not sexy.
>
> 2. Even in situations where mental illness or emotional instability may provide appeal, it is typically attached to costs not worth paying.
>
> 3. The idea that mental illness is sexy may have roots in harmful gender stereotypes.

Myth #38: "The More Emotional Intimacy, the Better"

When my patient Mark came to see me, he was experiencing issues in his marriage. He was in couples therapy and his wife complained that he needed to open up more. His couples therapist agreed that he had his walls up and encouraged him to explore his reasons for being emotionally distant in individual therapy. As I worked with Mark, it became clear that he felt that the purpose of his marriage was not to be super vulnerable and transparent. He was a traditional man and took a lot of pride in being a provider for his family, a dependable father, and a generous partner to his wife. His general stance was that marriage was not the type of relationship in which he could be completely raw and vulnerable with difficult emotions or challenges he was facing at work or in other areas of his life. He felt that he opened up enough and couldn't understand why his wife was not satisfied, because he had been this way for their entire relationship. They had been married for several years.

With Mark's permission, I was able to speak to his couples therapist. It's common for couples therapists and individual therapists to talk to each other with their patients' permission. Mark's couples therapist was able to facilitate a productive conversation between Mark and his wife about their differing relationship philosophies.

A relationship philosophy is built on a person's answers to questions like these: What makes a relationship work? Is it the quality of the emotional connection? Is it the feeling of always being on the same team? Is it passion? Is it building a meaningful life together and leaving behind a legacy? There are no right or wrong answers to these questions. What can happen in couples therapy is that people realize they have different relationship philosophies. In fact, there has never been, in my experience, a true 100 percent overlap between partners' relationship philosophies. Each individual in every couple needs to make some compromises to make the relationship work.

I am very fond of what the Gottmans' research has to say on this topic. For those of you who do not know, Dr. John Gottman and Dr. Julie Gottman have dedicated their lives to studying couples. With their method, they can predict, with high accuracy, whether or not a couple will get divorced after a single interview. Their insights have gifted couples therapists the Gottman Method; if the outcome of your relationship is not looking good, their interventions can help reengineer your dynamic so the relationship can be built to last. What they found is that approximately two-thirds of problems couples face do not have solutions.[1] When a problem in a relationship has a solution, then that solution should be implemented.

Often, the problems couples face come down to the advantages and disadvantages of the relationship itself. For example, if your partner is incredibly attractive, naturally extroverted, and very charming, they may get lots of attention from others when you two are at a social event. You may get jealous, insecure, and a bit possessive of them. That's normal. You cannot solve this problem. If you wanted to solve this problem, you would have to turn your partner into a completely different person. That's not advisable, because you don't want to throw the baby out with the bathwater. Instead, what the Gottmans recommend is that each member of the couple learn how to emotionally support their partner through an unsolvable problem. In this example, it can look like your partner giving you extra attention and affection when you get home after a night out.

To emotionally support your partner through your relationship's unsolvable problems, you have to be a little vulnerable. You can't receive emotional support if you can't share what you're feeling. In Mark's case, we were able to reach a compromise. I was sympathetic to his concern that he wanted to be "a husband to his wife and not like one of her girlfriends." That was the way he phrased it to me. He refused to entertain the idea that he should cry in front of her or direct genuine expressions of anger toward her, even if she made him angry. We were able to identify a middle ground. He could verbalize and articulate his feelings without revealing an expression of feelings that made him feel uneasy. Based on what I later heard from him and his couples therapist, his wife was fine with this idea and welcomed the change. She did not want him to come crying to her anytime there was a problem, either. She needed to feel closer to him in order to be a better partner and provide him emotional support when he needed it.

Here's the twist: As his individual therapist, I made no such agreement with Mark. If his wife really bothered him, he had full permission, from me, to express his feelings however he wanted to during the session. If he wanted to yell, he could yell. If he wanted to cry, he could cry. If Mark was preoccupied with fantasies of another life, where he wasn't married, where he was not tied down, where he didn't have the responsibilities of a father, he could talk about them out loud with me. It's not that Mark didn't love his family. But imagining how your life could have been different is completely normal. I actually think there's something quite reasonable and very loving about him never sharing those things with his wife or his children. If he was struggling in his sex life with his wife, he could think out loud about it with me, before bringing it to couples therapy. Mark, in all his stoicism and machismo, did individual therapy right when it came to aiding his journey in couples therapy.

When I became a therapist, I was surprised to learn that the most emotionally intimate relationships of my patients' lives would not always be with their partners; they would sometimes be with me or with other therapists. Therapy is a space where you can talk about anything, including the thoughts and feelings you have toward your partner that you would never share with them. And it's my job as a therapist to encourage you to emotionally open up even more, assuming that's clinically appropriate. For example, I have had survivors of sexual assault process their traumas with me who have been up-front in saying that they do not want their partner to know the details that I know. Their partners did not need to know the details in order to know that the traumatic event happened and what that meant for the survivors. If the survivors needed to talk about it in therapy, then they would talk about it.

When people are in the beginning stages of dating, emotional intimacy seems very desirable. It's exciting to feel called to share intimate details about yourself with someone you are falling in love with in the hope that they will become a special part of your life. It's normal to want to feel closer to the person you are getting to know. When people do that, when they open up, they are taking a risk. Being intimate, being emotionally close, means that you are risking hurt later. I am reminded of the book *Schopenhauer's Porcupines*.[2] Author Deborah Anna Luepnitz talks about how the porcupine offers the perfect metaphor for human intimacy. We want to be close to one another. In fact, we need to be close when storms come in life; and it doesn't matter who you are, storms always come. As we get closer, we risk accidentally hurting one another, in the same way porcupines that huddle together risk poking one another with their quills.

Lots of people have had the experience of opening up to someone and then later regretting it. That doesn't mean you shouldn't have opened up, but it does beg the question whether more intimacy is always better. In an age when Brené Brown made vulnerability cool and the Gottmans published research on emotional support, it seems the answer could be yes. There is even a trend on dating apps for people to not want to date others who haven't been to therapy, because not having been to therapy is thought to signal a barrier to emotional intimacy. I am not sure it's so simple. When it comes to professional relationships, more emotional intimacy is not always better, but the relationship can still be emotionally fulfilling. When it comes to friendships, emotional intimacy is not the only way to measure the value of a friend. For example, having common interests can lead to a fulfilling friendship even without emotional intimacy.

Intimacy is not good or bad. It simply is what it is. By keeping this in mind, you will be able to navigate relationships of all types and go at a pace that is appropriate for you.

> **3 THINGS TO REMEMBER ABOUT MYTH #38: "THE MORE EMOTIONAL INTIMACY, THE BETTER"**
>
> 1. Vulnerability is required in order to give and receive emotional support.
>
> 2. Emotional intimacy does not mean 100 percent transparency or expressing your emotions however you want.
>
> 3. Some relationships require less intimacy than others; they can still be fulfilling.

Myth #39: "Therapy Will Make You Ready for a Relationship"

I am learning the lessons of love just like everyone else. The longer I have been a therapist, and the longer I have been in therapy, the more I've noticed that many people want therapists to know something about love that most people don't know. For example, often someone will find out what I do and then ask me for advice about their dating life; or if I'm sharing a dating story that left me amused or bewildered, people may say something like "Obviously you get what's going on, given your job." I don't know about other therapists out there, but I find the journey of love just as confusing and exciting as anyone else does. Philosophers and artists have spent centuries trying to solve the mysteries of love, so I am not sure what unique insight or perspective mental health is supposed to have on the subject. The myth that therapy makes you ready for love, ironically enough, holds a lot of people back from finding love and meeting their special someone.

Psychobabble

The main issue is that people think that therapy will make them ready for a real relationship, but the most effective way to get ready for a relationship is to practice being in a relationship. Think about it: The first time you went on a date, you were probably not that great at it. Even if you are a natural-born dater, there were certainly things you could improve upon. After enough first dates, you get better at that stage of courtship. The first time you fall in love, it's a new and exciting experience that many people also find overwhelming. In fact, many people reflect on their relationship history and report that the "puppy love" they felt was actually infatuation, not real love. The real thing came later, as they got older and accumulated more experience. Additionally, sometimes people create an ideal version of themselves in their head, thinking that they need to be healed to a certain degree before they can properly engage in a loving relationship. Maybe that's true for some, but there are plenty of people with serious mental health conditions and childhood baggage who are in successful and committed relationships. I have treated many of them. The need to work on yourself does not preclude you from being ready for or deserving of deep and lasting love. I suspect that some people use therapy or their mental health as a way to bypass doing the work of practicing finding that special someone and successfully being in love.

Furthermore, talking about dating is very different from actively dating and talking to your therapist about it. The former has very limited utility; it would be like reading about mental health and then thinking you can easily facilitate a therapy session. Trust me, I read lots of books before I sat down with my first patient in my clinical internship. There are some things you just cannot learn about by talking or reading about them. You can only learn so much in medical school before actually practicing medicine, and there's only so much case law you can learn before you start to gain skill by actually trying a case in court. The part of your brain that understands something intellectually is different from the part of your brain that experiences that thing, particularly when it comes to deep emotional experiences like love.

Therapy can be helpful for developing certain tools or self-awareness to make you more skillful in dating or more resilient in the craft of romantic relationships. That said, I do not think it is wise to treat therapy as the be-all, end-all authority on the intricacies of love. If that were the case, more therapists would be in relationships the rest of us could look up to, and people would not spend a lifetime in therapy trying to sort out their dating lives. They would come to therapy briefly, learn the "answer" to their questions about love, and ride off into the sunset. That's not what I am observing when it comes to the relationships in my life or in my patients' lives, and that certainly has not been my experience. In my experience, nothing beats putting yourself out there and trying, learning, and growing. There's also biology and the dynamics of attractiveness, beauty, and sex appeal. Many people believe that there is a spiritual element to love as well. More logistical factors, including geography, technology, economics, culture, and age, also play a role. While you can discuss any or all these aspects of romantic relationships in psychotherapy, many of them are distinct from psychotherapy itself.

I am reminded of my patient Keenan, who came to therapy because he was struggling in the dating department. He described this experience of feeling super excited about someone he met, and then after a while, the "spark" would just die, along with any interest he had in continuing the relationship. Over the years, and with most of the women he dated, he would stay in the relationship anyway, diagnosing the sudden loss of interest as a problem with him and not his partners. Eventually, his partners would sense that something was off, and they would end up leaving him. Keenan couldn't blame them, but he was frustrated by how often this dynamic seemed to recur. As I worked with Keenan, I strived to instill deeper insight and engender a sense of self-awareness so he could better understand what was going on internally. We talked about his childhood. We discussed society's influence on men and their emotions, and we talked a lot about his feelings. We discussed his dating history in depth. We also talked about attachment styles, and that is when we started to make some progress.

Attachment styles have taken social media by storm. Some therapists and coaches build their entire brands by talking only about attachment styles and nothing else. Attachment styles are developed between children and their caregivers and can continue to play a role in the way individuals relate to others as an adult. There are two main attachment styles: secure and insecure. Insecure attachment styles are often labeled as anxious and avoidant. Sometimes people hyphenate attachment styles and add further distinctions—for example, "fearful-avoidant"—or talk about disorganized attachment or ambivalent attachment. I will focus only on secure, anxious, and avoidant attachment for simplicity. Here is how I sometimes talk about attachment styles to my patients:

> *Imagine a baby in a high chair who wants his mother's attention. The baby might make a fuss, and the mother will be there to talk to the child or get his sippy cup when he drops it*

on the floor. If the mother has to leave the room, the securely attached child knows the mother is eventually coming back. The anxiously attached child will cry and cry and will not stop until the mother returns. The avoidantly attached child withdraws inward, realizing that he should not rely too much on other people to get his emotional needs met. These patterns are styles for how we navigate the dilemmas of intimacy all the way into adulthood.

If someone's partner doesn't text them back, the securely attached person knows that the partner will when they have time. The anxiously attached person might follow up multiple times, fearful that something about the relationship is unstable. The avoidantly attached person will take the lack of communication as confirmation that they should keep love at arm's length. They might have thoughts like This is why you cannot get too close to others. It's much better to rely on yourself.

Dr. Stan Tatkin is the creator of the Psychobiological Approach to Couples Therapy (PACT) and is famous for introducing the metaphor of islands and waves to explain attachment styles. People who are anxiously attached are the waves. These people think something is wrong or they did something wrong when a person is not available to meet their emotional needs. The people who are avoidantly attached are the islands. They cope with relational stress through distance and self-reliance. When islands and waves fall in love, the waves will lap at the islands' shores as much as they can while the islands will float farther away toward the horizon. Mental health professionals sometimes refer to this as the anxious-avoidant trap.

Keenan resonated with the idea of being an island. At first, he resisted the interpretation, pointing out that he did not feel smothered or experience the need to isolate and self-soothe at the beginning of the relationship, before the spark died. This is the number one way people misunderstand and misuse attachment styles when it comes to understanding their dating lives. Attachment styles do not manifest until you become emotionally invested and attached to the other person. Sometimes the person is distant because they are just not that into you—that doesn't make them avoidantly attached. Sometimes that person who texts you multiple times in a row when you don't reply is just clingy or has poor impulse control. They're not necessarily anxiously attached, unless they developed feelings for you very quickly. In my experience, attachment theory is most useful when a relationship is already established, not in the early stages of dating.

When the spark died for Keenan, it was not the primary problem of his dating experience, but rather a symptom of his avoidant attachment style. He stopped letting himself be present and fully embracing the physical and emotional experiences of the relationship when things got too close. Keenan's strategy for navigating intimacy was to emotionally detach when he felt smothered. A big part of Keenan's journey was to become aware of this tendency, get curious about the underlying feelings, and develop different coping strategies. Instead of withdrawing, he would communicate that he needed a little space. Instead of idealizing a future girlfriend with whom the spark would never die, he practiced opening up to the person he was with at that time. He also gave himself permission to lose interest in someone if it turned out that the two of them were not compatible. That's not avoidant attachment. It's something that can happen over the course of a relationship, and that's okay, too.

One day, Keenan arrived in session and let me know he wanted to discuss ending therapy, at least for a while. Keenan explained that he felt he had benefited from therapy, but lately the sessions felt like catching up with a friend about his latest first date. He had the tools and self-awareness he needed to continue on the journey of love and felt it was more worth his time to focus on dating. If he met someone special and old patterns flared up again or he needed help, he would reach back out. I believe Keenan's perspective about how to use therapy as a tool to help him with his dating goals is exactly the right attitude. We could have continued to talk about how his past tied into his avoidant attachment. We could've examined other dynamics that were tripping him up about his dating life. But therapy is just one piece of the puzzle when it comes to finding and keeping love. Keenan understood that the insights he gained from therapy would be useless if he didn't apply them.

I think this is true not just for love, but for most or even all of the other ways psychotherapy can help you. The insights are useless unless you apply them to your life. That's the good news about the mental health field. You can be different. You can transform. Therapy can give you insight into how to go about doing so. My favorite psychological thinker is someone named Erich Fromm. Fromm was a very special thinker because, unlike Freud and Beck and so many other psychotheorists of his time, Fromm was not a medical doctor. He was a sociologist, so he conceptualized the psyche while considering the dynamics of history, capitalism, politics, and more. In his book *The Art of*

Loving, he describes love not as something you find or have or fall into, but something that you unlock within yourself.[1] According to Fromm, when you meet someone who takes your breath away in a way no one else ever has, it's not that they're *giving* you love that is more potent than anything else you've ever felt. It's more that *you* have unlocked a capacity within yourself to receive deeper love and passion than you ever had before. It's about you, not about them.

Everyone understands how true this is, because nearly everyone has had the experience of being closed off to love after a breakup and feeling open and desperate for love after being single for too long. According to Fromm, love is about practicing the craft of unlocking that capacity within yourself. That's why people look at therapy as the modern answer to all of love's problems. It's completely understandable that so many people are eager to see mental health or psychology as their answer to love-related questions. Relationships are emotional and confusing, and how we relate to people is clearly tied to our upbringing. But I have watched the most self-aware and talented psychological professionals I know still struggle when it comes to their love lives. If you struggle with dating or intimacy, remember that there is no replacement for opening yourself up to experiences of love and getting better at intimacy. If there's a mental health component or a mysterious emotional dynamic you cannot solve for yourself, therapy is a good stepping stone to help you get back on your way; therapy is not necessarily the journey itself.

As Fromm says in *The Art of Loving*, "It isn't a feeling, it is a practice." So get off the couch, and go practice. Your therapist will still be available if you need their support along the way.

**3 THINGS TO REMEMBER ABOUT MYTH #39:
"THERAPY WILL MAKE YOU READY
FOR A RELATIONSHIP"**

1. Therapy can be a useful tool, but it is not the only way to navigate love's problems.

2. Gaining insights about love in therapy is not the same thing as applying those insights to your life.

3. Love is not something you find—it's a craft and a practice.

Myth #40: "Using Therapeutic Language Makes You Emotionally Intelligent"

When I began treating Erika, her relationship was on the rocks. She spoke about communication issues and patterns in fights with her partner that made the relationship difficult to navigate. When I asked her for details about what the fights were like, she painted me a troubling picture. She explained that she tried her best to see her partner's side of things, but that if her version of reality ever conflicted with his, he would accuse her of "invalidating" him, "gaslighting" him, and "activating his trauma." Over time, she had grown quite frustrated, because she felt like she couldn't share her side of the story without being accused of causing psychological harm.

It became clear that the dysfunction in her relationship could not be solved just by working with Erika alone, so I referred her to couples therapy. In the meantime, I encouraged Erika to focus less on the actual definitions of *gaslighting, invalidation,* and *trauma*. Instead, I suggested, it would be best to focus on emotionally regulating herself, supporting her partner when she could, and repairing hurt feelings before sharing her side of the story. I hoped that this would allow Erika's partner to hear her better.

Like so many others, Erika was tempted to assume that her partner was automatically right just because he used therapy-speak. I assured her that she was allowed to disagree with him. She was as entitled to her version of events as he was, and a good couples therapist should be able to help them work through this. When I asked her about when he began using these terms, I was originally suspicious that he might have just started therapy. She explained that he wasn't in individual therapy at all. Erika noted instead that he spent a lot of time on TikTok watching mental health influencers and enjoyed many of the self-help pages on Instagram.

It's common for people to adopt therapy-speak when they begin their counseling journey. When people start going to therapy or learning about mental health, they acquire a new vocabulary with a lot of jargon. They assume that all these fancy new terms and their complex corresponding concepts make them more emotionally intelligent. Take it from a practicing psychotherapist: I have been fluent in therapy-speak much of my adult life, but I did not develop emotional sophistication simply because I acquired new vocabulary words. Instead, I had to learn how to integrate the awareness that therapy jargon gives me and apply it to different situations in the right way. Knowing the definitions of new words doesn't mean you necessarily have the insight to use those words correctly or understand how to apply the concepts.

Psychobabble

One year, during Thanksgiving, my family and I got into an argument. My brother and I wanted to go out for breakfast, but my mom feared this would spoil our appetites for an earlier Thanksgiving dinner. I don't remember how or why things escalated, but I was still in my first year of graduate school, and in my emotional overwhelm, I encouraged everyone to name their feelings and their conditions of satisfaction. Conditions of satisfaction are what a person wants and needs to feel like they have had a satisfactory experience. My suggestion was *not* well received. I remember my younger brother telling me to "stop talking like a goddamn therapist" because "it wasn't helping." I felt hurt by his response at the time, but looking back with hindsight and humor, it's *exactly* what I needed to hear.

Maybe my family could have benefited from pseudo group therapy that day, but no one wanted it at that moment. There were other ways to resolve the tension. I understood the terms I used, in contrast to Erika's situation. But I was using those terms to take control of the situation and assert myself as the more emotionally intelligent, levelheaded person. Even if Erika was an invalidating gaslighter, her partner's deployment of this language did not help their relationship. Erika's fights could have been processed without the psychological jargon. She could have been called selfish, inconsiderate, entitled, or some other word that would have helped me, as her therapist, better help her see how she was showing up in her relationship, according to her partner. In some ways, her partner's use of psychological jargon made my job harder, not easier, because he wasn't using layman's terms.

I have thought long and hard about why people find therapy-speak so alluring. One possible temptation for using therapy-speak is that it's an appeal to authority—a logical fallacy in which someone refers to reputation or expertise as the only or primary support for their argument, without providing any other evidence or reasoning. Perhaps it is easier, when in conflict, to use psychological jargon. After all, psychology apparently knows something essential about human beings. The problem is that psychology, like any other discipline, has its pitfalls. Psychology used to tell us that women became lesbians because they were envious of men's phalluses and that autism was caused by emotionally distant mothers. What psychological findings are popular today that we will look back on with embarrassment?

Toddlers call one another stupid heads, but people who spend too much time consuming mental health–related content often use the word *narcissist* very loosely. It appears to be an insightful and sophisticated slight, but in reality it is neither—and using the word this way is unfair to the survivors of narcissistic abuse. If you use therapy jargon as an appeal to authority, I hate to break it to you, but it doesn't necessarily make you seem emotionally intelligent.

Another reason that using mental health language is so attractive is that it can be very effective in morally justifying whatever it is you're arguing for. Part of the reason, as David Brooks has argued in *Bobos in Paradise*, is that we live in a society in which health has replaced morality as the standard for goodness. Today, Brooks observes, people talk about "the things that are forbidden [as] unhealthy or unsafe. The things that are encouraged are enriching or calorie burning. In other words, we regulate our carnal desires with health codes instead of moral codes."[1] Have you ever noticed this? People will justify making certain choices and cite their mental health as an adequate justification. For example, deciding to cut off a family member is stripped of any moral or ethical implications when your mental health is on the line. In today's world, we judge cigarettes because they cause cancer, not because nicotine is a vice. We judge junk food because it's metabolically unhealthy, not because you are indulging in gluttony for eating it. As mental health becomes more in vogue, there is a great temptation to use therapy-speak less as a tool for explaining reality and more as a tactic for justifying what we believe to be right or wrong.

These trends are not without real risks. The only thing more concerning than my patients' loved ones hurling therapy-speak-related accusations was how quickly my patients internalized those labels. Once I had a consultation with a man who was concerned he was a narcissist because, after his son was born, he mistakenly thought he would be able to go to the gym in his usual routine and leave his wife at home with the baby. Was she in the right to feel angry that he was leaving her at home, without considering that she would be in charge of childcare on her own? Sure. Did what she said to him warrant his reaching out to a therapist to rule out a narcissistic personality disorder diagnosis? I don't think it did. Lots of men have struggled with adjusting to fatherhood long before therapy-speak took hold of culture, and something tells me that lots of men will continue to struggle.

If you use therapy-speak to convey emotional intelligence, then consider this: Learning therapy-speak is a bit like learning to play an instrument. You probably can't learn it well completely on your own, and you will almost certainly need someone with education or experience to teach you. When you start, you will be confined to rigid chords and notes. After a while, when you're more practiced, you can riff to your own tune and add your own style.

For example, when you start learning about mental health, you may be confined to rigid ways of thinking and speaking: for example, "I hear that you're feeling _____." (Note the "I" statement combined with use of the active-listening skill to foster a sense of empathy.) Over time, you can better showcase your emotional intelligence by combining that practice with your personality. How would I say that to my loved one and some of my patients? I would not say, "I hear that you're feeling sad." I might say, "Dude, I totally get it. That sounds like a total bummer!" In this way, I take my knowledge of "I" statements and reflective listening and put it in *my* voice. If I can do so at the right time and in the right way, I am taking my knowledge and insights about mental health and applying them effectively. As you can see, accomplishing this takes much more than simply knowing the definitions of certain terms. It requires time, practice, empathy, and humility.

As the years have gone by and my therapy skills have sharpened, I have learned that there's a big difference between talking like a therapist, on the one hand, and utilizing my knowledge of human emotion and behavior to skillfully navigate conflict while speaking like nobody but myself, on the other. In my opinion, every therapist worth their salt knows how to take their knowledge of psychology and apply it to their conversations. They also know that we often need to be careful before using diagnostic psychological language.

My advice to everyone is to be careful when leveraging therapy-speak against people in your life. It may provide a brief authoritative flair but will not necessarily lead to productive dialogue or any sort of lasting relational cohesion. Also be careful when leveraging therapy-speak against yourself. As someone who is basically fluent in therapy-speak, let me tell you, it doesn't always make my personal journey easier. It allows me to intellectualize a lot of nonsense that my own therapists usually have to dig me out of just so I can see the truth, which was usually obvious all along. Whenever you can, keep it simple. Use ordinary language whenever ordinary language will suffice. And when it comes to being emotionally intelligent, show, don't tell.

> **3 THINGS TO REMEMBER ABOUT MYTH #40: "USING THERAPEUTIC LANGUAGE MAKES YOU EMOTIONALLY INTELLIGENT"**
>
> 1. Therapy jargon is not usually helpful in interpersonal conflict or when describing subclinical (nondiagnostic) experiences.
>
> 2. We already have plenty of ordinary words to describe a wide variety of complex human experiences, and these are often more descriptive and less fraught.
>
> 3. If someone uses therapy jargon as an appeal to authority, they don't sound more intelligent. Whenever you can, show, don't tell.

Acknowledgments

Writing this book would not have been possible if it were not for all the support I received along the way. The first thank-you goes to my family. Thank you to my mom and dad for raising me to be outspoken and brave, as I would surely not be so comfortable putting my ideas out into the world if you hadn't instilled a sense of resiliency. Thank you to my younger brother for always being there for me. Thank you to my grandmother, Barbara, for instilling a love of reading and writing at a young age.

Thank you, Abby Skeans, Branden Polk, and Jason Cavnar, for being so encouraging and loving as I find my path both professionally and in life. Thank you, Jenn Sherman and Sara Battista, for being my work wives and allowing me to rant and complain about anything and everything. Thank you to Charm Augustin and Cara Winslow for allowing me to focus on the creative work that I enjoy most. Thank you, Manuela Welton, Krista Kleiner, Amanda Cole, Jenner Deal, John Markland, Andrew Nguyen, Dr. Kevin Jardine, and all those who have supported my pursuit of a career in media. Thank you, Jonathan Merrit, for believing in

Acknowledgments

this project, and thank you, Angela Guzman, for seeing the vision when so many others did not.

A big shout-out to Dr. Kate Maloney, who put me on a path to become both a psychotherapist and a content creator many years ago. Thank you to my graduate school professors at Northwestern University, specifically Dr. Jinah Rordam and Dr. Russell Fulmer; you were formative in my development as a practitioner. A special shout-out to Dr. Michele Kerulis for assisting me with the writing process and being a valuable second pair of eyes. Thank you, Courtney Fraser, Dr. Barbara Brown, and Dr. Simona Efanov, as my formative clinical training has set me up for success throughout my private practice career thus far. Thank you to Alex Harrison, Dr. Steven Lazarus, and Dr. Ben Smoak for providing me with valuable supervision and training; your wisdom echoes throughout the pages of this book. Thank you to Professors Donald Moon, Indira Karamcheti, Jon Cutler, Gil Skillman, and Cecilia Miller at Wesleyan University; each of you helped me hone critical thinking skills and a writing style that will continue to serve me for the rest of my life and career.

It's perhaps most important to thank my patients. I am constantly reminded that I have the most privileged job in the world when you let me into your lives, your minds, and your hearts. You all help me believe in the potential of the mental health field each time you bravely take a step forward. My advocacy for the mental health field is fueled by each and every one of you.

I also want to thank my followers on social media. This book is written for you, and it is also your support that made this book possible. In a lot of ways, being called an influencer doesn't make sense to me. I do not see myself as "influencing" anyone. I had no

Acknowledgments

idea how many people were hungry for a conversation about the nuances of mental health terminology and discourse until you all helped me see that. I view my work less as a way to influence you and more as a way to be a platform and conduit for your passion and endless curiosity for a field we all love so much. Thank you.

Finally, a big thank-you to New York City and all my friends and acquaintances who reside here. You provide me with endless inspiration, stimulation, and community. I could not have written this book anywhere else.

Notes

Introduction: The Tower of Psychobabble

1. Rebecca Jennings, "When TikTok Therapy Is More Lucrative than Seeing Clients," *The Cut*, May 17, 2024, https://www.thecut.com/article/tiktok-therapy-money.html.
2. Jonathan Sperling, "Mental Health Is Costing the US Economy Billions—Increasing Access Could Be the Solution," *Business & Society*, May 28, 2024, https://leading.business.columbia.edu/main-pillar-business-society/business-society/mental-health-cost.
3. Jennifer Bronson and Marcus Berzofsky, "Special Report: Indicators of Mental Health Problems Reported by Prisoners and Jail Inmates, 2011–12," US Department of Justice, Office of Justice Programs, June 2017, https://bjs.ojp.gov/content/pub/pdf/imhprpji1112.pdf.

Myth #1: "Everyone Should Go to Therapy"

1. Jenny Mollen, *I Like You Just the Way I Am: Stories About Me and Some Other People* (New York: St. Martin's Griffin, 2015).

Myth #5: "Personality Frameworks Are Reductive, Inaccurate, and Not Helpful"

1. Gary Chapman, *The Five Love Languages* (Chicago: Northfield Publishing, 2010).

Notes

Myth #7: "Receiving a Diagnosis Is Terrible"

1. Mary C. Zanarini, Frances R. Frankenburg, John Hennen, D. Bradford Reich, and Kenneth R. Silk, "Prediction of the 10-Year Course of Borderline Personality Disorder," *American Journal of Psychiatry* 163, no. 5 (May 2006): 827–32, https://pubmed.ncbi.nlm.nih.gov/16648323/.

Myth #8: "Mental Health Diagnoses Are Just Made-Up"

1. David Dobbs, "What Is Mental Illness? A Peek Through the Murk," *Wired*, May 18, 2011, https://www.wired.com/2011/05/what-is-mental-illness-a-peek-through-the-murk/.
2. G. Eric Jarvis, Laurence J. Kirmayer, Ana Gómez-Carrillo, Neil Krishan Aggarwal, and Roberto Lewis-Fernández, "Update on the Cultural Formulation Interview," *Focus: The Journal of Lifelong Learning in Psychiatry* 18, no. 1 (January 24, 2020): 40–46, https://www.ncbi.nlm.nih.gov/pmc/articles/PMC7011218/.
3. "Ludwig Wittgenstein," *Stanford Encyclopedia of Philosophy*, last updated October 20, 2021, https://plato.stanford.edu/Entries/wittgenstein/.

Myth #9: "Your Diagnosis Is Your Identity"

1. Taylor Tomlinson, *Look at You*, Netflix, https://www.netflix.com/title/81471774.

Myth #10: "You Can Diagnose Yourself"

1. Anthony Yeung, Enoch Ng, and Elia Abi-Jaoude, "TikTok and Attention-Deficit/Hyperactivity Disorder: A Cross-Sectional Study of Social Media Content Quality," *Canadian Journal of Psychiatry* 67, no. 12 (2022), https://journals.sagepub.com/doi/full/10.1177/07067437221082854.
2. Diego Aragon-Guevara, Grace Castle, Elisabeth Sheridan, and Giacomo Vivanti, "The Reach and Accuracy of Information on Autism on TikTok," *Journal of Autism and Developmental Disorders* (August 6, 2023), https://pubmed.ncbi.nlm.nih.gov/37544970/.

Myth #11: "Everyone Gets Depressed and Anxious"

1. Nick Haslam, "Concept Creep: Psychology's Expanding Concepts of Harm and Pathology," *Psychological Inquiry: An International Journal for the Advancement of Psychological Theory* 27, no. 1 (2016), https://www.tandfonline.com/doi/full/10.1080/1047840X.2016.1082418.

Notes

2. Yu Xiao, Naomi Baes, Ekaterina Vylomova, and Nick Haslam, "Have the Concepts of 'Anxiety' and 'Depression' Been Normalized or Pathologized? A Corpus Study of Historical Semantic Change," *PLOS One* 18, no. 6 (2023): e0288027, https://pubmed.ncbi.nlm.nih.gov/37384729/.
3. James Patterson, *Grand Expectations: The United States, 1945–1974* (Cambridge: Oxford Univ. Press, 1997).
4. Abraham Maslow, *Toward a Psychology of Being*, 3rd ed. (New York: Wiley, 1999).
5. Allen Frances, *Saving Normal* (New York: William Morrow, 2013).
6. Lauren J. Harvey, Fiona A. White, Caroline Hunt, and Maree Abbott, "Investigating the Efficacy of a Dialectical Behaviour Therapy–Based Universal Intervention on Adolescent Social and Emotional Well-Being Outcomes," *Behaviour Research and Therapy* 169 (October 2023): 104408, https://www.sciencedirect.com/science/article/pii/S0005796723001560.

Myth #12: "The Reason You Can't Focus Is ADHD"

1. Casper-Gallup, *The State of Sleep in America: 2022 Report*, accessed December 16, 2024, https://www.gallup.com/analytics/390536/sleep-in-america-2022.aspx.

Myth #14: "Your Awkward Friend Is Neurodivergent"

1. JewishCare NSW, "Brave Talks: Judy Singer, Pioneer of the Global Neurodiversity Movement," YouTube, December 8, 2022, https://www.youtube.com/watch?v=LDOQxduRbQs.
2. Judy Singer, *NeuroDiversity: The Birth of an Idea* (Cambridge: Oxford Univ. Press, 2017).
3. Autism Speaks, "Early Start Denver Model (ESDM)," accessed December 16, 2024, https://www.autismspeaks.org/early-start-denver-model-esdm.

Myth #16: "Boundaries Are Just Preferences"

1. Brighter Sex, "Brené Brown: Boundaries," YouTube, September 12, 2020, https://www.youtube.com/watch?v=TLOoa8UGqxA.
2. Esther Perel, "Establishing Boundaries," *MasterClass*, accessed December 16, 2024, https://www.masterclass.com/classes/esther-perel-teaches-relational-intelligence/chapters/establishing-boundaries.
3. The Holistic Psychologist, "A Beginners Guide to Setting Boundaries," YouTube, May 12, 2019, https://www.youtube.com/watch?v=tUOvY6LfmlA.

Notes

Myth #17: "People Gaslight You When They Disagree"

1. Sam Cabral, "Gaslighting: Merriam-Webster Picks Its Word of the Year," *BBC News*, November 29, 2022, https://www.bbc.com/news/world-us-canada-63798242.
2. *Merriam-Webster Dictionary*, "gaslighting," accessed December 16, 2024, https://www.merriam-webster.com/dictionary/gaslighting.
3. *Merriam-Webster Dictionary*, "gaslighting."
4. David Foster Wallace, *Authority and American Usage* (New York: Little, Brown and Company, 2006).

Myth #18: "Your Ex Is Definitely a Narcissist"

1. Ramani Durvasula, *It's Not You: Identifying and Healing from Narcissistic People* (New York: Penguin Random House, 2004).
2. TEDx Talks, "Narcissism and Its Discontents: Ramani Durvasula, TEDxSedona," YouTube, January 28, 2019, https://www.youtube.com/watch?v=aHHWgG7dB6A.
3. Allen Frances, *Saving Normal* (New York: William Morrow, 2013).
4. DoctorRamani, "The Best Way to Deal with Narcissists Without Arguing," YouTube, November 6, 2022, https://www.youtube.com/watch?v=O4otiLhz0Qg.
5. The Diary of a CEO, "The Narcissism Doctor: '1 in 6 People Are Narcissists!' How to Spot Them & Can They Change?," YouTube, February 29, 2024, https://www.youtube.com/watch?v=hTkKXDvSJvo.
6. The Diary of a CEO, "The Narcissism Doctor."
7. Alice Miller, *The Drama of the Gifted Child* (New York: Basic Books, 2008).
8. Nancy McWilliams, "Some Thoughts About Schizoid Dynamics," *Psychoanalytic Review* 93, no. 1 (February 2006): 1–24, https://www.proquest.com/docview/195088140?sourcetype=Scholarly%20Journals.

Myth #20: "Everyone Has Trauma"

1. Robert Sapolsky, *Why Zebras Don't Get Ulcers*, 3rd ed. (New York: Holt Paperbacks, 2004).

Myth #21: "Trauma Is the Same Thing as Grief"

1. George Bonanno, *The End of Trauma* (New York: Basic Books, 2021).
2. *Dietrich Bonhoeffer Works*, vol. 8, *Letters and Papers from Prison* (Minneapolis: Fortress, 2009), letter no. 89, page 238, https://www.thegospelcoalition.org

/blogs/justin-taylor/bonhoeffer-on-why-god-does-not-fill-the-emptiness-when-a-loved-one-dies/.

Myth #24: "Questioning Trauma Discourse Harms Survivors"

1. Carol Tavris and Elliot Aronson, *Mistakes Were Made (but Not by Me)*, 3rd ed. (New York: Mariner Books, 2020).
2. Joe Nucci, "Is the Word 'Trauma' Overused?, featuring Matthias J. Barker, Therapy vs. the World," YouTube, April 29, 2024, https://www.youtube.com/watch?v=LxTy-QkF1i0&list=PL2IJNtlAaQCeWeCpsUaRNF-Z6iGczcB07&index=11.

Myth #25: "Your Mental Illness Is a Systemic Problem"

1. Ferdi Botha and Sarah C. Dahmann, "Locus of Control, Self-Control, and Health Outcomes," *SSM—Population Health* 25 (November 24, 2023): 101566, https://www.ncbi.nlm.nih.gov/pmc/articles/PMC10698268/#:~:text=Locus%20of%20control%20describes%20the,et%20al.%2C%202020.

Myth #26: "People Aren't Evil, They're Just Mentally Ill"

1. TEDx Talks, "The Most Important Lesson from 83,000 Brain Scans: Daniel Amen, TEDxOrangeCoast," YouTube, October 16, 2013, https://www.youtube.com/watch?v=esPRsT-lmw8.
2. Richard Gonzales, "Researcher Says Aaron Hernandez's Brain Showed Signs of Severe CTE," *The Two-Way*, NPR, November 9, 2017, https://www.npr.org/sections/thetwo-way/2017/11/09/563194252/researcher-says-aaron-hernandez-s-brain-showed-signs-of-severe-cte.
3. Bob Hohler, "Aaron Hernandez's Brain Was Severely Afflicted by CTE," *Boston Globe*, November 9, 2017, https://www.bostonglobe.com/sports/patriots/2017/11/09/doctor-details-her-findings-after-examination-aaron-hernandez-brain/USjpN1t5Ic02JPG20heeVN/story.html.
4. Kimberly Gorgens, "Traumatic Brain Injury in Criminal Justice," University of Denver, accessed December 16, 2024, https://psychology.du.edu/tbi.
5. Anna-Karin Ångström, Anneli Andersson, Miguel Garcia-Argibay, Zheng Chang, Paul Lichtenstein, Brian M. D'Onofrio, Catherine Tuvblad, Laura Ghirardi, and Henrik Larsson, "Criminal Convictions in Males and Females Diagnosed with Attention Deficit Hyperactivity Disorder: A Swedish National Registry Study," *JCPP Advances* 4, no. 1 (January 20, 2024): e12217, https://acamh.onlinelibrary.wiley.com/doi/full/10.1002

Notes

/jcv2.12217#:~:text=Crude%20estimates%20for%20the%20full,compared%20to%20individuals%20without%20ADHD.

6. Noman Ghiasi, Yusra Azhar, and Jasbir Singh, "Psychiatric Illness and Criminality," *StatPearls* (March 30, 2023), https://www.ncbi.nlm.nih.gov/books/NBK537064/#:~:text=The%20public%20perception%20of%20psychiatric,violent%20crime%20than%20the%20perpetrator.
7. P. Räsänen, J. Tiihonen, M. Isohanni, P. Rantakallio, J. Lehtonen, and J. Moring, "Schizophrenia, Alcohol Abuse, and Violent Behavior: A 26-Year Followup Study of an Unselected Birth Cohort," *Schizophrenia Bulletin* 24, no. 3 (1998): 437–41, https://pubmed.ncbi.nlm.nih.gov/9718635/#:~:text=Men%20who%20abused%20alcohol%20and,crimes%20than%20mentally%20healthy%20men.
8. Hung-En Sung, "Alcohol and Crime," *Blackwell Encyclopedia of Sociology*, first published August 1, 2016, https://onlinelibrary.wiley.com/doi/10.1002/9781405165518.wbeosa039.pub2.

Myth #27: "Mental Health Education Is Always Beneficial"

1. Darby Saxbe, "This Is Not the Way to Help Depressed Teenagers," *New York Times*, November 18, 2023, https://www.nytimes.com/2023/11/18/opinion/teenagers-mental-health-treatment.html.
2. Abigail Shrier, *Bad Therapy: Why the Kids Aren't Growing Up* (New York: Sentinel, 2024).
3. Victoria M. E. Bridgland, Payton J. Jones, and Benjamin W. Bellet, "A Meta-Analysis of the Efficacy of Trigger Warnings, Content Warnings, and Content Notes," *Clinical Psychological Science* 12, no. 4 (August 18, 2023), https://journals.sagepub.com/doi/10.1177/21677026231186625.

Myth #30: "Therapy Is Not Political"

1. Nili Solomonov and Jacques P. Barber, "Conducting Psychotherapy in the Trump Era: Therapists' Perspectives on Political Self-Disclosure, the Therapeutic Alliance, and Politics in the Therapy Room," *Journal of Clinical Psychology* 75, no. 9 (September 2019): 1508–18, https://onlinelibrary.wiley.com/doi/abs/10.1002/jclp.22801.
2. Stock Analysis, "Talkspace Market Cap," accessed December 16, 2024, https://stockanalysis.com/stocks/talk/market-cap/.
3. Reina Gattuso, "Therapy Is Political. It's High Time Therapists Acknowledge This," *Talkspace*, November 18, 2020, https://www.talkspace.com/blog/mental-health-is-political/#:~:text=%E2%80%9CA%20lot%20of%20therapists%20might,collective%20bodies%2C%E2%80%9D%20said%20Woodland.

Notes

4. "Reina Gattuso," *directory*, City University of New York Graduate Center, accessed December 16, 2024, https://www.gc.cuny.edu/people/reina-gattuso.
5. American Counseling Association, *2014 ACA Code of Ethics*, accessed December 16, 2024, https://www.counseling.org/docs/default-source/default-document-library/ethics/2014-aca-code-of-ethics.pdf?sfvrsn=55ab73d0_1.
6. Derald Sue and David Sue, *Counseling the Culturally Diverse* (Hoboken, NJ: Wiley & Sons Inc., 2016).

Myth #32: "Therapists Should Never Give Advice"

1. Jonah Hill, *Stutz*, Netflix, November 2022, https://www.netflix.com/title/81387962.

Myth #36: "Your Date Is Love-Bombing You"

1. Anna Gionet, "The Love Bombing Survey," *Love & Relationships*, Shane Co., May 10, 2022, https://www.shaneco.com/theloupe/jewelry-education/love-relationships/love-bombing-survey/.

Myth #37: "Freak in the Head, Freak in the Bed"

1. Jessica Taylor, *Sexy but Psycho: How the Patriarchy Uses Women's Trauma Against Them* (London: Constable, 2022).

Myth #38: "The More Emotional Intimacy, the Better"

1. Zach Brittle, "P Is for Problems," The Gottman Institute, last updated October 30, 2024, https://www.gottman.com/blog/p-is-for-problems/.
2. Deborah Anna Luepnitz, *Schopenhauer's Porcupines* (New York: Basic Books, 2002).

Myth #39: "Therapy Will Make You Ready for a Relationship"

1. Erich Fromm, *The Art of Loving* (New York: Open Road Media, 2013).

Myth #40: "Using Therapeutic Language Makes You Emotionally Intelligent"

1. David Brooks, *Bobos in Paradise: The New Upper Class and How They Got There* (New York: Simon & Schuster, 2010).

About the Author

Joe Nucci, LPC, is a licensed psychotherapist, writer, and social media influencer. His content contextualizes mental health misinformation, pop psychology facts and fallacies, and culturally misconstrued ideas. Joe's work focuses on empowering individuals—whether or not they have a background in psychology—so they can live a life with greater a sense of agency and self-awareness. You can find his writings in his newsletter and his content at @joenuccitherapy. Visit joenuccitherapy.com for more.

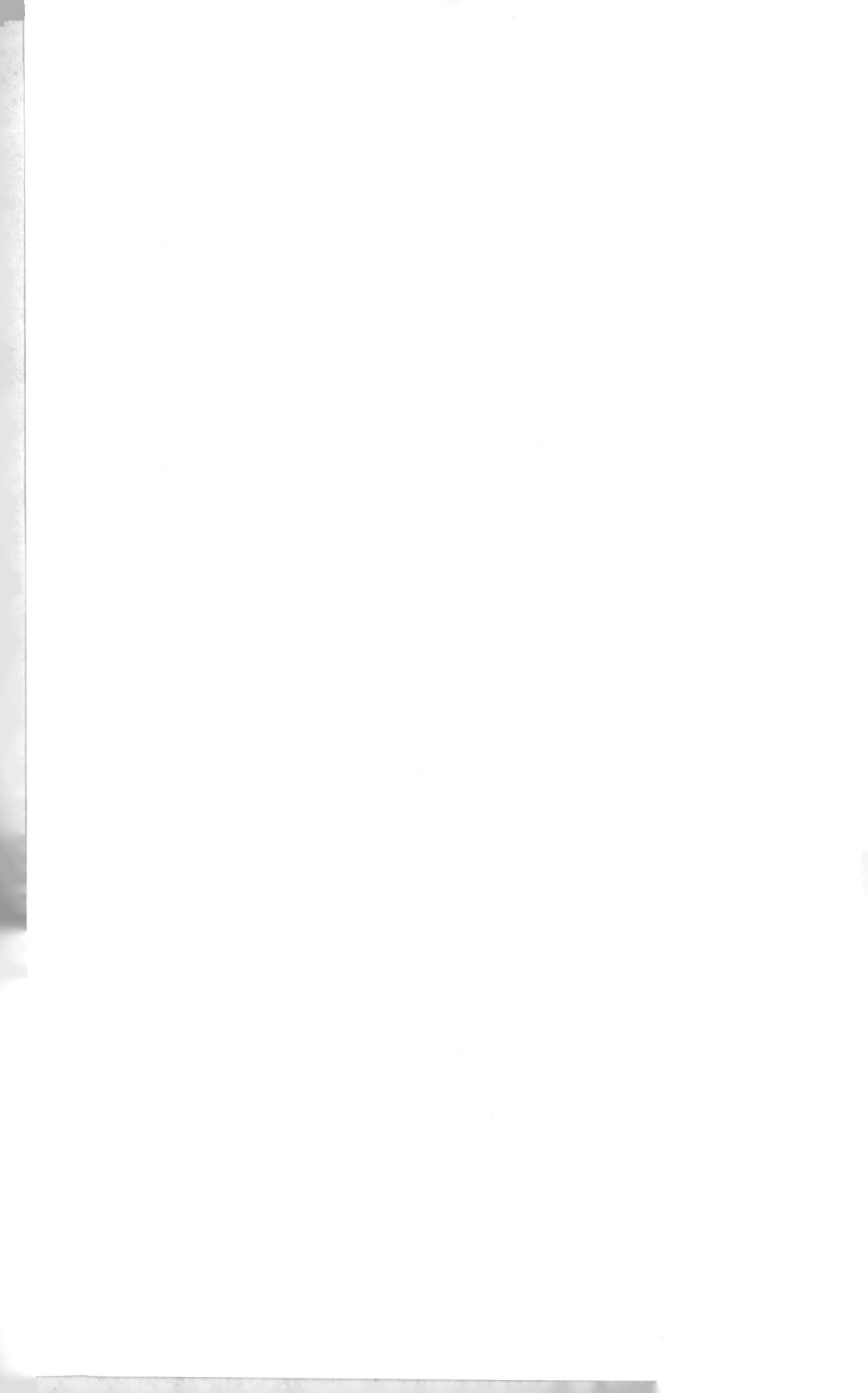